PRAISE

DIARY OF A MED STUDENT

DIARY

OF

A

MED

STUDENT

DANIEL AZZAM

AJAY NAIR SHARMA

COPYRIGHT

DISCLAIMERS

The views and opinions expressed in this book are those of the individual story authors and do not necessarily reflect the position of any of the Editors.

All patient, doctor, school, and hospital names were changed to protect the anonymity and confidentiality of the subjects of the story. Any matches in names or initials are entirely coincidental.

ISBN 978-1-0879-0697-3

www.diaryofamedstudent.com

FOUNDERS & EDITORS-IN-CHIEF

Daniel Azzam

Ajay Nair Sharma

FACULTY ADVISOR

Johanna Shapiro, PhD

CREATIVE WRITING EDITORS

Peter Azzam, MD

Shankar Iyer, MD

Carina Mireles-Romo

Kaosoluchi Enendu

Hayoung Youn

Howard Chang

Jacob Stultz

Manali Sapre

Nikhil Bellamkonda

Shonit Nair Sharma

TECHNICAL SKILLS TEAM

Jenny Torres | Timothy Vu | Elsa Li

CONTRIBUTING MEDICAL SCHOOLS

Albany Medical College

Albert Einstein College of Medicine

Baylor College of Medicine

Brody School of Medicine, East Carolina University

California University of Science and Medicine

Carle Illinois College of Medicine, University of Illinois

Carver College of Medicine, University of Iowa

City University of New York School of Medicine

Drexel University College of Medicine

Eastern Virginia Medical School

Frank H. Netter School of Medicine, Quinnipiac University

Geisel School of Medicine, Dartmouth University

Geisinger Commonwealth School of Medicine

Harvard Medical School

Icahn School of Medicine, Mount Sinai

Indiana University School of Medicine

Johns Hopkins University School of Medicine

Keck School of Medicine, University of Southern California

Lewis Katz School of Medicine, Temple University

Loma Linda University School of Medicine

Max Rady College of Medicine, University of Manitoba

Mayo Clinic School of Medicine

Medical College of Georgia

Medical College of Wisconsin

Northern Ontario School of Medicine

Pacific Northwest University College of Medicine

Paul L. Foster School of Medicine, Texas Tech University

Perelman School of Medicine, University of Pennsylvania

Renaissance School of Medicine, Stony Brook University

Rosalind Franklin University of Medicine

Sanford School of Medicine, University of South Dakota

Sidney Kimmel Medical College, Thomas Jefferson University

State University of New York Downstate College of Medicine

Stritch School of Medicine, Loyola University

TCU and UNTHSC School of Medicine

The Ohio State University College of Medicine

Tufts University School of Medicine

University of Alabama at Birmingham School of Medicine

University of Arizona College of Medicine, Tucson

University of California, Davis School of Medicine

University of California, Irvine School of Medicine

University of California, Los Angeles School of Medicine

University of California, Riverside School of Medicine

University of California, San Diego School of Medicine

University of California, San Francisco School of Medicine

University of Central Florida College of Medicine

University of Colorado School of Medicine

University of Florida College of Medicine

University of Illinois College of Medicine

University of New Mexico School of Medicine

University of South Carolina School of Medicine

University of Washington School of Medicine

University of Wisconsin School of Medicine

Yale School of Medicine

To

MEDICAL STUDENTS
and your stories worth sharing

*Medical school can be trying, frustrating, and downright
difficult at times. If you ever feel the need to talk to
someone, we encourage you to speak to your loved ones,
your school administration, or professionals for help.
You are not alone in this journey.*

CONTENTS

FOUNDERS' NOTE

For two months on our Internal Medicine rotation, we arrived at the hospital bright and early, spending the next 12-16 hours completing tasks ranging from the menial to the critical. When we finally returned to our apartment as roommates, we had barely enough time to scarf down dinner, take a shower, and complete one practice question to feel some semblance of productivity. We were exhausted most evenings, but with one conversation, our excitement returned.

"You won't believe the day I just had!"

Each night, we would share a story of what happened to us in the hospital. Often, it was something hilarious. Occasionally, it was something tragic. And other times, it was simply something amazing. Our tales of humor, sorrow, joy, and inspiration became as much a staple of our rotation as rounding, noon conference, and sign-out. We couldn't wait to hear what kind of adventure the other got into that day.

When we shared these stories with our classmates, we were met with hearty laughs and stories in return. We weren't surprised our classmates had equally memorable tales, we were just elated by their desire to share their personal experiences. To all of us on rotation, this was therapeutic. A way for us to commiserate on the life of a third year. To acknowledge that it was okay not to be perfect. To recognize that we were not alone.

Diary of a Med Student is a testament to these stories. After receiving over 200 submissions from over 50 medical schools, this book truly represents the voices from students across nations. Not just from third year, but from all years. Not just from our school, but from all schools. It is a book created by medical students, for medical students, doctors, pre-med students, and their loved ones to look backward, forward, and laterally on the wonderful world of medical school. This book offers a space to reflect on our emotions, process their meaning, and share them from the perspective of medical students writing in a diary.

By capturing these historic tales of medical training during a global pandemic, social unrest, and economic insecurity, we believe that this book represents a diverse collection of unifying tales that provide optimism in a time of need. We hope that reading these relatable, emotional tales is unifying and comforting. Let this book spark a powerful domino effect in changing medical education, creating a safe space for inner reflection and expressing emotion, to ultimately enhance physician wellness.

Daniel   *Ajay*

PREFACE

The authors have done a masterful job of engaging medical students from 54 different schools to assemble *Diary of a Med Student*. More impressive, perhaps, is they accomplished this while enduring a global pandemic and social upheaval surrounding the systemic racism and inequities present in society today.

I have to admit, the book brought back fond memories of my own medical school days and the requisite copy of *House of God*, which I dutifully read over and over in the 1980s. Certainly, those of us who have the benefit of a few years of experience on these young authors have been guilty of extolling our own tales from our early days of training. Something about the mix of idealism, an insatiable desire to learn, and the time to actually talk to and observe patients makes our medical students the ideal group to observe the humanism inherent in the healthcare environment.

The unjaded views of some of life's most joyous, funny and tragic moments are relatable to all who have walked before the authors. And, the grouping of the stories into sections titled Humor, Sorrow, Joy and Inspiration is an ideal way to organize the 101 stories. At the end of the day, health care is about our patients and their loved ones, and the degree of empathy apparent in many of the stories recognizes the relationships that our students have made with their patients. These connections are vital to the evolution and training of all medical students on their path to becoming caring and compassionate doctors.

Congratulations to these talented students for brightening our days.

Michael J. Stamos, MD, FACS, FASCRS
Dean, School of Medicine
University of California, Irvine

FOREWORD

"Do I even belong here?" I pondered to myself as everyone turned in their exams, and I was still only a quarter of the way through. I remember stepping out of the lecture hall and listening to everyone talk about the tougher questions – somehow the ones I had trouble on were obvious to the majority. I put in my best effort consistently, and I was still far behind. Later I'd find out my score, and I was not surprised at the lackluster performance. Medical school was no joke.

I had this same feeling when I got to college at USC. I didn't go to the same high school these other kids did. Where I went, 20% of students dropped out by senior year. My new peers went to schools where 20% went to top colleges. I somehow found a way to get through it, and felt like I almost snuck into medical school at UC Irvine. I remember wondering how I even got into a school in California. Now the bar was even higher, that this imposter had somehow joined the class.

These exams continued to drag on throughout MS1 and MS2, yet I could not crack the code. No matter how many hours I put in, what advice I took, what study techniques I tried, I just could not figure it out. There was too much new information and I had a hard time getting it to stick. The "drinking water out of a fire hydrant" analogy would haunt me...it was actually true and I hated it.

I would study with Andrew Berg all the time, and when we would get into study delirium, we would start drawing pictures on paper and on a random whiteboard we recovered from the sidewalk outside. This was really just desperation – the exam was tomorrow, and we still had a ton to learn. How do we condense this and remember it?

You have all been there. When you are wired on caffeine (or your drug of choice), are suffering from lacking sleep, and have been trying to cram as much information as you can into your head for God knows how many hours, and you know that no matter what, you have to perform the next day. It's in situations like this where you either rise above it or fail. I failed, a lot, but now, something finally clicked. We were flowing. We were creating the most ridiculous drawings, symbols, and characters to quickly get through and represent all the remaining study material. Strep agalactiae was naturally a baby in space, and on the exam, I just had to go back into space and answer the question without even trying. It felt good, I was finally figuring medical school out.

After using these techniques to get through more and more exams, we had some validation that we had stumbled upon something great. This simple, and even fun study technique enabled me to go from the struggling hopeless medical student, to someone who could keep up with the class. We would run through drawings with our friends, and they would swear by them. Around this time, we realized one of our classmates, Bryan Lemieux, was also a great artist and believed in the idea. Even though we were still students at the time, we decided we wanted to share this even more broadly. It was too special to keep among ourselves. We had that feeling of excitement you get when you find something really cool and you just have to share it. We had a vision of medical students from all over world learning from us the way our friends and classmates were learning from us. We wanted to not only recreate this learning experience, but also the experience of joy when you finally feel like you can handle medical school. The feeling that you do belong. The feeling that you did not get here by accident.

The Sketchy seed had been planted in our minds, and we have worked tirelessly to bring that vision to life. The path to where we are today has been an absolute rollercoaster. Throughout the course of going through medical school, residency, and building a product and company at the same time, I have gone through many emotions – including joy, sorrow, humor and inspiration. It is these feelings that give our memories life. No journey is void of them, and if there is one thing I have learned in all my experiences, it is that we must embrace these feelings. It's okay to feel them, and what matters is accepting them and continuing forward. That is what drew me to this book.

Though we all have a unique journey, we will all go through the same mix of feelings in different ways. We are all feeling them, even if we don't show it. I am sure some of you have felt the same feelings I have shared in my story. *Diary of a Med Student* helps removes the veil. It gives us all an opportunity to read the stories of our colleagues in training and experience their feelings with them. It helps us understand that we are not in this alone, and we are all more connected than we may think.

Saud Siddiqui, MD
Co-Founder, SketchyMedical

BLACK LIVES MATTER

Life can only be understood backwards;
But it must be lived forwards.
— Søren Kierkegaard

DIARY OF A MED STUDENT

PART ONE

—

TALES

OF

SORROW

—

Tears are words that need to be written.
— Paulo Coelho

Give sorrow words; the grief that does not speak knits up the o-er wrought heart and bids it break.
— William Shakespeare

Our greatest joy and our greatest pain come in our relationships with others.
— Stephen R. Covey

NANCY

"Sorry, that was our last roll." The sales associate's voice echoed through the empty grocery store. I sighed, feeling the warm moist air reverberate from the mask back to my cheeks.

The town felt somber on my drive home, but it was almost noon. It was when Nancy would come by and drop off our mail with her glistening smile. Nancy was more than our mail-person. She was there for life's most important moments, letters from my dad across the world, the day I got my first work check mailed, and the day I got accepted to medical school.

That memory, I recall vividly. "It's a thick one, it isn't thin," she laughed as she squeezed the letter and left it at the screen door last fall. It was from my dream medical school. She waved as she ran off our porch and across the yard to our neighbor, the leaves crunching in her wake.

"I got in!" I exclaimed to her the next morning as she handed me the mail. She knew every Wednesday that November, I would already be waiting on my porch for her arrival. We hugged. "I guess I won't be seeing you next Wednesday then," she chuckled. "I hope not!" I joked.

Fall passed and winter came and with that, coronavirus. It was as if everything in the world had stopped, except Nancy. I turned off my Zoom camera and walked to the door. "White Coat might be canceled," I announced through the window. She felt my defeat through the door. "Don't let this get you down. We need people to keep going—people to heal," she comforted. Her smile beamed through her N95 mask.

Spring came. Nancy delivered my stethoscope one warm April day. After laying it on the porch, she trudged across the lawn hunched over. I saw Nancy less and less. Distracted by my anxiousness about school, April passed. May arrived.

"Where's Nancy?" I asked my mom, feeling guilty for not checking in. She had not come by in weeks. "She's at the community hospital." Our town had been hit hard by COVID-19. "There's a letter in the mail for you, but no return address," my mom continued, handing over a wrinkly pink envelope doused in Lysol.

"This pandemic will pass, but you must go on. When the world is sick, we need hopeful healers." It was from Nancy.

Nancy perished a week later due to complications related to coronavirus. More than an essential worker, she was part of the fabric of our suburb, interwoven in our everyday life. She connected loved ones across the world by postal mail. Despite rain, snow, or a pandemic, she was there for our community.

She was truly a healer to me.

A MOTHER'S CRY

When a trauma comes to the hospital, everyone's pagers ring simultaneously. It sounds almost synchronous. Yet, there is an eerie feeling as the room falls quiet and everyone urgently reads their pagers.

Today's message: 12-year-old motor vehicle accident, head strike, unstable, med flight, arrival in 15 mins.

We are prepared for traumas. When a child is involved, it is always emotional. As soon as I was able to scrub out of the OR, I heard the helicopters landing on the rooftop. My cue to run to the ED.

On arrival, the room was full of roughly 20 physicians and nurses and eerily quiet. I edged my way to the front where I found my team. My colleague debriefed me: 12-year-old male with autism, car vs bike, flew 40 ft, no helmet, head strike, loss of consciousness, non-responsive, med flighted from Maine, mother in-route.

I gulped as I glanced over at the paramedics wheeling in a young boy, covered in tubes, lying motionless. Our chief resident commanded the code and the ED hustle and bustle commenced.

Neurosurgery scrubbed in and decompressed the skull to relieve intracranial pressure. Everyone fell into their roles, but this all ceased when we heard the loudest, shrill cry come from the entrance. His mother arrived.

She was dressed in work attire and inconsolable. People cleared a path for her to see her son. She whispered, "I love you and I need you to come home." I looked around the room where eyes were sunken, heads were low as if everyone felt her pain. I lifted her off the floor and walked her through the next steps. "His skull was decompressed to relieve pressure; he is now going to the OR to take a flap of the skull off to maintain low intra-cranial pressure and to fix the multiple broken bone. You can come with us but will have to wait outside when he enters the OR. She nodded. The hospital became a one-way street leading to the OR. Outside of the OR, she was told to say her goodbyes.

These words to him would be her last. She forgave him for taking his bike without her permission, for not wearing his helmet and told him that she loves him more than anything she has ever loved.

When the news was delivered, the pain echoed down the hallways. This type of pain was worse than the previous cry. This cry was naïve to my ears. It came from a place only a mother crying for her child would understand. The hospital fell quiet. But just as it always does, the hustle and bustle would slowly return.

HEART OF A LION

"In the jungle, the mighty jungle, the lion sleeps tonight..."

A tear rolled down my cheek as I listened to the music playing overhead. I had to remind myself not to wipe it because I was fully scrubbed in the OR, meaning there was an invisible barrier at the level of my chest that marked the border of the "sterile field" that my hands were confined to remain below. Before me was the body of a little girl who had been hit by a car the night before. Though her brain had been irreparably damaged, her heart was still beating – I knew this because I was looking right at it, bouncing so vigorously that I was afraid it would literally bounce right out of her chest and onto the floor of the OR.

This was my first ever organ procurement. It was at once the most tragic and spectacular thing I have ever experienced in my life.

Earlier that morning, a transplant attending, fellow, resident and I, a third year medical student, had all piled into a private jet to fly hundreds of miles to join teams of doctors who had come from around the country to harvest organs for their patients.

Before the procurement began, the whole team listened to a note written by the donor's parents. They wrote about their daughter's joyfulness and spirit in life, and how even in death they felt she would have wanted to pass on a chance at a new life to others. Altogether, six strangers from across the country would have something in common tomorrow thanks to this one girl's sacrifice – one heart, two kidneys, the liver would be split in half, and a small intestine. The parents also mentioned in their note that their daughter loved Disney music. In her honor, her favorite Disney songs were played in the OR throughout the entire procedure.

I was blown away by the magnitude of this human endeavor. Hundreds of people had come together at a moment's notice to make this possible – doctors, nurses, transplant coordinators, the ambulance driver and jet pilots, and so many others behind the scenes, working tirelessly to save the lives of strangers they would never meet. But above all, I was moved to tears by the compassion of her parents. Their little girl had been stolen from them with unimaginable cruelty not even 24 hours earlier. But even in a moment of unfathomable grief, they had chosen generosity.

Even in her last moments, it was clear for all to see that this little girl truly did have the heart of a lion.

A MOMENT

"You're SO lucky...I would give anything to be you right now," my patient's grandma said to me as I anxiously sat between my patient's knees preparing to birth her great-grandson. She and six other family members were in the birthing suite, eagerly awaiting the arrival of the newest member of their clan.

Just two months into my clinical rotations, as an MS2 aspiring to become an OB-GYN, this exact moment was a dream come true – the chance to deliver a real BABY.

My attending was at my side, instructing me through each step. I followed the directions to a tee. There was no way I was going to mess up this moment.

"Just one more push! We see the head! You're so close, PUSH!"

My adrenaline was sky-high. A thousand thoughts raced through my mind, yet I was still focused on making this delivery go smoothly.

Next thing I knew, the baby's head had fully emerged. My attending swiftly guided my hands through external rotation, delivery of the anterior and then posterior shoulder, and then...

My first delivery!

My patient and her family cheered and cried tears of joy as she held her baby – after nine months, the moment they had waited for was finally here.

But this perfect moment was cut short as the Peds team swooped in for the routine newborn evaluation. Or so we thought.

My patient bled heavily after delivery, so my attending told me to begin uterine massage as the team checked on the baby.

"Is my baby going to be okay?" my patient asked me. Her eyes were wide with fear as tears streamed down her face. While continuing to massage her uterus, I said, "Your baby is in good hands, the doctors are making sure that your baby is okay."

My attending came back with somber eyes and told the new mother that her baby was having difficulty breathing and that CPR was being performed.

"I will check on the baby and update you as I receive more information," my attending told my patient. As my attending left the room, my patient began to sob uncontrollably. I too, felt a wave of worry come over me.

As soon as my patient's bleeding stopped, the nurses took over, and I anxiously rushed out to check on the baby.

In the newborn nursery, I saw panicking providers huddled around the crib, doing everything in their power to make sure this new life would live.

The EMTs had arrived, prepared to airlift the baby to the nearest tertiary care center. The lead EMT walked over to the crib. The Peds resident had been doing CPR for 30 minutes.

"It's time to call it," said the EMT.

"Time of death. 8:52 p.m.

LUCKY

It's 5:30pm, and I'm finishing up my last note, growing aggravated by the lagging computer and the fact that I have been at the hospital for over 12 hours. As a medical student with no designated workplace, I am using a computer on wheels in the hallway, easily distracted by the voices in passing.

One voice, in particular, grabs my attention.

It is a female voice on the phone. She is talking to a family member, possibly her mother.

"Call his brothers, he is dying!" She exclaimed.
"I don't care if they haven't spoken in years and hate each other, my dad is dying, call his family!"

Over-hearing this heartbreaking conversation, I could not stop my gaze from shifting towards this voice. I glanced at her, and I immediately recognized her.

We went to high school together. She sat behind me in history class for a whole year. Though we weren't particularly "close," I would call her a friend.

I tried to keep from staring, but eventually she caught my glance.

After she finished her phone call, she approached me with a gentle smile.
"How are you doing?" She asked.
"I didn't know you went to school here, lucky you!"

As much as I wanted to reply with the same question, "How are you doing?"
We both knew the answer.

As our conversation ended, I felt my eyes well-up with tears. My current concern was finishing up a note on an outdated computer. Hers was watching her father pass away before her eyes.

With long work days and sleep deprivation, we often forget who we are working hard for, writing notes for, staying late for.

It is for our patients.
It is for their families.
It is in the hopes of providing care and comfort during one's darkest, most difficult times.

It is not a burden.
It is a privilege.

She is right.
Lucky me.

SILENCE

The clock read 3:30 AM on the final night of my OBGYN night-rotation. Three mothers required emergency C-sections that night, and we shared two ORs and one anesthesiologist with another team.

Sarah was one of the mothers awaiting an operation. Her baby was diagnosed with Osteogenesis Imperfecta, a disease that left the baby with bones that cracked like dry twigs at the slightest pressure. Sarah knew her baby would not survive, but she wanted to have a chance to hold her child once while his little heart was still beating. However, as the night deepened and other mothers delivered before Sarah, the barely perceptible heartbeat of Sarah's baby quieted until only Sarah's heartbeat remained.

At 3:30AM, Sarah was brought to the OR, loss hanging in the air like a miasma. Upon feeling our touches, Sarah began to cry. Her murmurs of "I can't do this" crescendoed into gasping cries. Sarah's husband clutched her hands and brought his face to hers, forming a private space between the two as they remained surrounded by masked and gowned strangers. As Sarah calmed, my fellow took a breath to steady herself, her voice clear when she finally said, "Scalpel."

Abdominal incision. Fascial layer. Rectus muscle. Layer by layer, we moved closer to Sarah's baby. Uterine incision. The first glimpse of the baby, five little toes. When Sarah's baby finally entered the world, he did so in silence. A silence so profound and final that it deafened everyone standing in the OR. A silence that spoke to how far we have come in medicine, but how far we have yet to go.

ROCKSTAR

Her infectious laughter was just one of many beautiful things about MK. At age 14, she was a caring older sister to six, with dreams of becoming an electric guitar playing entrepreneur. From her hospital bed, MK successfully launched her own handmade jewelry business. While my biggest worry at age 14 was the state of my acne, MK was so mature in her determination that she never allowed anything to become an obstacle in pursuing her dreams.

The program was intended to assign the perfect pairing - and to my luck, the intent matched reality. The day I met MK, she was in excruciating pain and before I could say hello, she told me to go away. The next day was filled with awkward conversation, which she blatantly pointed out. And then, we clicked, like friends effortlessly do.

"Rebirth." That is how MK referred to her bone marrow transplant. That day, she wore her shaven head with such confidence, rightfully claiming her rockstar status. From then, she spent weeks in the same hospital room, which meant more time with me. We spent hours playing UNO, creating a handmade blanket, watching Netflix and Disney movies, dancing to songs, talking about boys in her class, and laughing through it all. We spent so much time laughing about the silliest things. She once named her IV pole after the boy she was crushing on (whose name shall forever remain a secret). When I think of her, I picture her carefree belly laugh. Here is a teenage girl undergoing immunosuppressive therapy, constantly being poked and prodded, missing school, her friends, her siblings and still, she is flashing her bright smile and laughing with me. She had the unique ability to find joy in the present and extend that joy to others.

Second year of medical school swooped in, consumed my attention and blurred my priorities. Despite being there for many dim days, despite holding her hand while she was too ill to speak, watching her struggle with physical therapy, seeing the skin changes, the weight loss, I had not even considered her death. How does anyone comprehend that a 14-year-old rockstar could die?

In rockstar fashion, she left me desiring more time, but grateful for the beauty she brought to my life. I think of her often, but particularly during church or when Sickle Cell Disease or Graft-versus-Host disease is discussed. I am a better friend for the remorse I feel for not being there enough. I will be a better physician, and human being, because of the kindness and patience she modeled.

AN EMPTY SEAT

A month into medical school, we received an email informing us our families wouldn't be able to join us during White Coat. Our school's auditorium was too small. The entire class was disgruntled and upset, some going to great lengths to try to somehow get their families in for this momentous occasion. I, however, was slightly relieved. I knew, that even if permitted, the only person I cared to see there would never show up.

"You're gonna fix my heart when you become a doctor right?" My mother used to remind me daily as a child. Just the idea that I, someday, would have the potential to heal her and many others was comforting to her. She strived for me to be the best I could be and I wouldn't be where I am today without her.

It was her dream to see me graduate from medical school, sacrificing her own well-being, since the day I was born, to give me the tools I needed to be successful. It was debilitating when she passed away before I even got accepted into medical school.

"What's the point?" I thought, "this was all for nothing." Why wear a white coat if she never got the chance to see it on me?

But then, I remembered what she truly wanted, what she sacrificed everything for. It wasn't to make her proud, or to post my accomplishments on social media. It was for me to be the best I could be, and to 'fix' people. So, I continued on for her. I donned that white coat in her honor, knowing that, regardless of the size of the auditorium, there will always be an empty chair on this day, and every occasion after. But she will forever be with me, pushing me to be the best I can be.

GRAB MY HAND

My morning coffee was just beginning to kick in as I sat down at a workstation in the cardiac ICU. It was my first day rotating with anesthesia, and a brief tour of different IV lines had just flown right past me.

"Yo! I never thought I'd run into you, it's been ages!" someone whispered loudly.

My eyes lit up with surprise as I recognized the voice. My longtime classmate and teammate on the soccer field was walking towards me; we hadn't seen each other in at least 6 years. We started to catch up and I realized that he was working with the care team for the patient I was about to see.

"So have you cared for this person before? How have things been?" I inquired, in an attempt to better understand the patient's hospital course. I listened as he started to explain the patient's admission to the hospital: "He has a complicated seizure disorder and had been riding his bike on a trail when he suffered a seizure. He's been here for-"

"CAN YOU GRAB MY HAND." A woman's voice interrupted with impressive volume, causing both of us to look immediately at who she was speaking to.

I stared in disbelief at the scene – the woman, a neurologist, was assessing my patient's neurological function. The patient looked around my age, if not younger than me, and holding his hand was his mom, who reminded me of mine. As the neurologist bellowed louder, my friend and I grew more silent.

My mind sunk into the gravity of the situation, overcome with a sense of sorrow. The patient and his mom, both in age and physical appearance, shared an uncanny resemblance to my life. So much so, that I felt guilty for what seemed like even existing in the same space as them both.

As I began to step into the shoes of the mother and child, my guilty glances of pity transformed into something more – to a truer kindness seeing through the eyes of empathy.

"That could have been me... it seems like mere circumstance," I couldn't stop thinking to myself, glancing from my computer towards the patient each time I did.

A STRANGER

Last Saturday, I arrived at the hospital at 7 AM for my weekend shift. Our team received a new patient first thing in the morning, a woman with metastatic breast cancer presenting with hemoptysis. The overnight resident warned us she might decompensate at any moment.

At 7:30 AM, she started hemorrhaging into her lungs, but she was still herself – a person who had lived 77 years, had come to the hospital with her husband, and had entrusted us with her wishes amidst the flurry of the unknown. Despite the fact that she may have recognized the severity of her condition, she was someone who expected to see her family the next day. Most of all, she was still very much alive.

By 8:30 AM, she was actively dying. She became unresponsive, body turning white, heart rate dropping. My residents were still rounding on their other patients, but I had finished rounding on mine, so I stood. I stood watching the telemetry monitor at the nurses' station, my heart plummeting every time her heart rate dropped past 40, down to 0, back up to 20, and teetered on the edge of life. I stood there knowing that her husband was a few yards away from me in her room, sobbing silently. I wanted to walk into the room and hold his hand, but faced with this intimate moment, perhaps the most intimate of all moments, my legs turned to iron, so I stood.

Before long, the telemetry line went flat. My team handled the situation well – they comforted her family and made medical choices based on the patient's wishes. But the moment passed, and the team continued, moving onto the next task on the to-do list. I didn't know the patient, I don't even remember her name, but when I got home I cried. I cried again writing this, harder than I did the first time.

It is strange to occupy a world in which death becomes part of your workflow. I'm sure that there will be patient deaths that sadden me deeply, and others that feel like there is one less patient on my list to worry about, as foreign as that seems now as I mourn the death of this stranger. Maybe becoming desensitized, at least partially so, is necessary - to carry the weight of all our patients' suffering would be too consuming. Or maybe I'm wrong – maybe I will come home and cry often, not just for deaths but for unfortunate diagnoses or mistakes I have made. It's difficult to decide which outcome I'd prefer – to feel more professional, more balanced, or to feel more like most other people, those who are deeply struck by the fragility of life and death.

TODAY'S THE DAY

"Today's the day I'm going to die." She said.

"Excuse me?" I asked.

"I woke up today with a feeling that it's going to be my last day," she said.

This was not how I thought the end of my morning would go. It was a relief to be on heme consults and stroll in at 8am, but since there were still no new consults, and I was bored of UWorld questions, I decided to say "Hi" to my patients from when I was on the oncology service last week. The one I was most eager to check on was diagnosed with stage 4 lung adenocarcinoma.

When I first met her, she was frail and breakable, and too consumed with pain to even look up. Slowly, over the week, with pain medications and our other interventions, she was able to open her eyes. She even smiled with them. No longer writhing in pain, she opened up to me. She told me about her children, her unborn grandchild and how she loved making pasta sauce for her family. She knew whatever she had was bad, but that she was going to survive it. By the end of that week, she was the one reassuring me.

This morning, however, there was no reassurance. She opened her eyes and looked at me with fear and helplessness, took my hand and said, "Today's the day I'm going to die."

I paused.

I had known when patients were going to die before, but they were never the ones telling me that themselves. Do I tell her nurse? Call my fellow? Call a code?

Instead, I squeezed her hand back and calmly said – the truth is I don't even remember what I said to her. I just remember feeling terrified that this lady, with the warmest of eyes, was going to die today.

Later that day, I discussed the encounter with the oncology fellow and asked if she thought the patient might actually die today. She smiled, as if this were a typical question, and said the family had decided on a rehab facility since she was stable for discharge. Two weeks later, she told me the patient was seen in clinic and doing well.

I often wonder why she greeted me with those words that day. Maybe it was her impending discharge to an unknown place, the fear of her new diagnosis or all of the uncertainties she now faced.

I don't know if she's still living today, if she'll get to see her grandchild or make pasta sauce again.

I do know that I'll never forget the terror I felt that day and realize that it was nothing compared to the fear and uncertainty she was facing, despite her outward appearance and objective data claiming her wellness.

Sometimes, all we can do is squeeze their hand back.

DEAR JOHN

Dear John,

To refresh your memory, I was the medical student on the palliative care team who visited you often during your hospitalization, expecting a joke each time I entered the room. I would enter with the goal of tackling a difficult end-of-life issue, but more often than not, you deflected with a hilarious corny joke.

I came to enjoy visiting you – not to accomplish anything in particular, but to laugh and be present for you and your wife. I remember fondly us asking the nurse if she was aware of the "EGG" (electrograstrogram) procedure ordered for the day and her confusion as to what that meant and her reaction of rolling her eyes when she realized we were not talking about an egg. Although you were faced with a terminal cancer diagnosis and given months to live, you always had a joke ready for me.

Except when you didn't. Just a day earlier, you had been jovial and full of life. But the next day, I did not see the usual spark in your eyes. For the first time, you looked like how you sounded on the medical record: an old man with terminal cancer who was wasting away from lack of nutrition.

I remember how shocked I was at how quickly the disease took its toll. That day our team signed off from following you daily. I remember each morning for the following week I would look up your file on the computer to see you were still in the hospital and if any complications had happened. I still feel guilt when I think about how, at the end of each day, after I had finished my duties with my patients and was faced with the decision to go home or come check in on you, I chose to go home.

I don't know why I did that. Maybe I wanted to remember you as the guy who kept his humor and good nature in the face of suffering and not as a withering cancer patient. Although now I feel selfish and cowardly. I wish I had come to visit you. You have probably passed away by now but I wish you knew the impact you had on me. It was an honor to have shared some of your last days with you.

Thank you.

PEDIATRIC BLUE

When the news came, I was in the middle of helping my attending place a femoral line.

"Doctor, we just got a call." A nurse had poked her head into our room. "You have a pediatric code blue coming in."

A pediatric code blue? My gloved hands shook a little, covered with blood from our line placement attempts. This was just my fifth day of clinical rotations. I was rotating in the emergency department, and today I was assigned to the critical care team.

We reentered the ED just as the code blue rolled in from the ambulance. For a moment, I couldn't process what I was seeing: a LUCAS device was strapped on the stretcher, the force of its compressions buckling the patient's chest like plastic. But this was not a manikin, this was someone barely younger than myself — someone fighting to come back to life.

The trauma room filled with activity: EMS relayed information to our staff, my attending ran over with an ultrasound, nurses readied pushes of epinephrine. Somehow, I ended up at the head of the bed, a bag valve mask in my hands.

"Med student, give ventilations." The words came from somewhere in the room, and I let adrenaline guide my movements. Breath, 2, 3, 4, 5, 6. Breath, 2, 3, 4, 5, 6.

Those few minutes of ventilating were the most challenging experience of my medical education to date. The plastic airways of practice dummies were much easier to ventilate than this patient's, who had chest damage from LUCAS and blood bubbling up the ET tube with every breath I gave. I wondered, Am I hurting him?

The patient's family was brought in just before we called off compressions. Eyes all throughout the room were glistening: the family's, a nurse's, an EMT's, mine. After they left the room, compressions were finally called off. LUCAS stopped, leaving behind just heavy silence.

Afterwards, I went immediately to lunch and lingered there for an hour, trying to regain enough composure to step back out into the Emergency Department and face the rest of the day. I had expected to experience a patient death during my rotations, but I had never thought to encounter one so early. However, I want to remember the emotions of that experience forever. I want to remember my sadness, the calmness of my attending, the connectedness I felt with the other healthcare workers working with me, the raw human emotion that permeated the room. This experience was difficult for me in many ways, but I hope that the memory of it serves to mold me into a stronger, more caring physician.

COMPRESSIONS

I heard the pagers go off and felt a rush of adrenaline as we bolted toward the hospital, trying desperately not to roll an ankle in my Danskos. Arriving, amidst the commotion, I noticed his wife in the corner and felt a pang of remorse. I remembered that this was a husband, a father, an uncle. I recalled my role. Forcing gloves on my sweaty hands, I took my place in line. I remembered what I had read in House of God: "Rule number 3: at a cardiac arrest, the first procedure is to check your own pulse." Instinctively, I felt for my radial pulse. My heart rate had almost tripled. Deep breath.

Two excruciatingly long minutes. I recalled past boxing matches, where rounds of 90 seconds felt like an eternity, but the stakes were nowhere near as high. I felt my glasses falling off my nose, sweat beading on my forehead, blood rushing into my cheeks. I knew that his circulation depended on me, so I kept going.

10 minutes later, resuming CPR, I felt his hand on my arm. I looked down at his face, his unmoving eyes, seemingly unaware of the bodies around him, poking him, compressing his heart. It felt like he was weakly trying to push me away, like I was hurting him. I really felt like I was hurting him; I couldn't get over that. I finished my round, but I did not go again.

Instead, I watched the CPR stop. I watched his wife walk to his side and pour her heart out in their last minutes together. I heard her cry and her anguish and her love. I walked out to let her be with him and just him while he passed. I hastily wiped the tears from my eyes. I got a hug, a pat on the shoulder. I heard the pager go off again, and we rushed downstairs.

ISCHEMIA

Her toes were black. Burnt to a crisp although they were not warm. In fact, they were stone cold - like death. While her toes were still attached to the remainder of her body, they were no longer a living part of her. The oxygen she inhaled with each breath would never reach them. So while it may have been difficult for her to wrap her mind around the idea that within the hour, her foot would be amputated - severed just above the ankle - this was in fact old news to the rest of her body.

I was a first year medical student and had just walked into the Emergency Room for my first 'preceptor' visit. "Oh boy do we have something good for you," my preceptor announced as I walked into the sterile, fluorescent room. Coincidentally I was coming from a lecture on the complications of type 2 diabetes so the mechanism behind this peripheral neuropathy was fresh.

The only operation to salvage her foot would involve creating a bridge between the healthy vessels of her foot and the dead vessels of her toes. However, the vascular surgeons had already determined her vessels were too small to perform this bypass. We were simply waiting to see if her living tissue could reperfuse any additional regions of her foot, allowing the surgeons to salvage more of her limb during the amputation procedure.

Death does not normally work in such a slow, methodical manner. It most often takes a person all at once. In this particular situation, I was watching death take Mrs. Ramirez, inch by inch. With every passing moment, the black boundary between necrotic tissue and pink flesh slowly crept up her foot. It was as if the grim reaper was attempting to tuck her in, but struggled to get his cold blanket past her toes.

MR. BKA

A man from the department of corrections presented for a vascular surgery consult. He had a wound on his foot, obtained from poorly fit shoes he continued to wear. To me, that is why he came, a wound. A wound that could be dressed, perhaps debrided and maybe even amputated if necessary. In my young hopeful medical student mind, he would be leaving soon afterwards.

It all started with the wound. The wound turned into debridements. The debridements turned into a below knee amputation (BKA). Then came the acute kidney injury on top of his previous renal transplant. From there came the GI bleeding, the metabolic derangements, the hypoxemic respiratory failure. The ICU transfer. The intubation. I'd listen anxiously with my eyes squeezed shut when code blue was called, his new room number memorized in my head.

He was a man of flat affect. He answered only "yes" or "no" and did not deviate from those responses. He didn't say thank you, please wasn't mentioned, and never gave a smile. So why was I still looking over his chart now in his ending days with a pit-in-my-stomach feeling?

Maybe it's because he came in shackles with guards at his bedside. It kept me awake at night that we couldn't tell his family when I started to see a decline. Maybe it's because we are supposed to advocate even harder for those who can't or won't advocate for themselves. Or maybe it's because I felt guilty that perhaps even I was treating him differently because he was a prisoner. After he was transferred to the ICU, I'd walk by his room to see what kind of state he is in. And even after, I sat at a different hospital, continuing to follow him "peripherally."

He's at the end now. And it all started with a wound.
Poorly fitting shoes. Something that seems so small is
now the end of a life.

Nursing told me he said, "I won't be going back to
prison" when he found out about the discharge plans.
Never before have I see the human body crumble at the
hands of the mind. At the hands of giving up, not
wanting to live anymore, not fighting anymore.

Medicine hurts. I think it's supposed to. We are
supposed to advocate so strongly for our patients that
their losses sometimes end up as our losses too. If you
take the humanity and love out of medicine, it all
becomes algorithms. We lose sight of what our patients
need from us. I know that this is only the beginning of
the hurt I feel for my patients, but I accept it with my
vulnerable human being open arms - and fall into the art
that is medicine.

PATIENT UNKNOWN

I was a sub intern on my neuro ICU elective when I first encountered a patient's name listed as "unknown" in the EMR. The patient had been "found down" on the street after suspected opioid overdose. In the neurologic ICU, he was essentially brain dead, save an intermittently reactive pupil which we treated as needed with mannitol. Any attempts at saving this man's life or recovering brain function would be futile. However, he had no advance directive, and with no name to go on initially, no surrogate decision makers could be found.

After calling around, we finally found a name reached his halfway house, but still could not track down any family members. After further detective work, we discovered the contact information of two of this man's close friends at the halfway house.

We discussed the ethical dilemma of the situation to the friends. Both independently said that the patient would not want futile extensive measures. Given the unconventional nature of the situation, we set up a meeting with the hospital's ethics team to ensure our approach was reasonable. Our team's perspective was that it was cruel to keep this patient alive with no potential of brain recovery, and we had found two people who were close to the patient who confirmed he would not want any extraordinary measures. The ethics committee agreed that this was a responsible approach.

As we got ready to withdraw life-sustaining care, I remember thinking to myself that I did not want this poor man to die alone. Even though he was not conscious of anything, it still felt important to me that someone was there who knew him and cared about him.

I think if I was in that situation, I would want a friend or loved one there, even if I didn't know they were there.

We got ahold of the two friends again, told them the plan, and offered them a chance to come say goodbye. They both without hesitation came the next day. One of the men stood quietly in the corner, forcing back tears. The other man stood at the patient's bedside, looking forlornly at his friend.

I suppose the reason this patient stuck with me so much is that he made me think about death in ways I never had before. In the end, I was proud that my team was able to give this patient a "compassionate death," surrounded by people who cared about him.

WE DIDN'T KNOW

"We didn't know."

This week we've had lectures, small group sessions, & standardized patient interviews focused on substance abuse. This is a complex, emotional topic for me.

Two different physician instructors commented on their education on & history of prescribing opioids. This was the first time that I've heard a physician frame this issue in a way that pulled some culpability away from patients.

Just 10-15 years ago, physicians were taught that "Pain is the 5th vital sign." Many physicians believed it was acceptable/safe to liberally prescribe opioids, and that one would be remiss in not utilizing them for pain. "We didn't know"...that the actions of well-meaning physicians would contribute to what is now an epidemic.

My mom struggled with opioid addiction for most of my life. She had a complicated relationship with doctors. She felt unheard and helpless. She questioned how drugs designed to ease pain could be ruining so many lives.

Before the reckoning of the Sackler family, my mom used to call companies like Purdue Pharma "criminal." But how on earth could SHE contribute to a change in health policy? Who would listen to a recovering addict with a long criminal record related to drug abuse?

As a future physician, I am left with questions. That sometimes we might hurt patients in order to adapt? That we are beholden to our patients? That we should listen when a patient says "something isn't right"? I'm not sure. But I do know that if my mom were alive today, she would be more at peace that this discussion exists.

CIRCLE OF LIFE

Performing my abdominal exam in Gynecologic Oncology clinic, I thought, "There is the liver's edge. Wow, I'm good." What were those nodules though? I did not have enough time to peruse her chart; the clinic day was too packed. "It has to be cirrhosis from her Hep C."

How obviously wrong I was. This woman, who happened to have metastasis from a cervical malignancy, was succumbing to the nasty crab itself: cancer.

I quickly pulled up the patient's recent CT scan. There were about 100 metastatic sites in her liver – I was deflated. The nodules I was so confused yet excited to have discovered were nothing but the finish line for a young woman's life. How could I have been so enthusiastic to have palpated the liver when such malignancy was present?

Only a matter of minutes had passed, but I knew a very difficult discussion was going to follow. With our attending, the next 40 minutes was filled with tears from not only the patient and her daughter, but me. I had no connection to this patient. Why did I hurt?

Our attending initiated the conversation by being honest about the failure of chemo to the spread of her disease; concluding with the topic of hospice. "How much time, doc?" said the patient. "Months."

I could feel the gravity of the situation. This patient now knew her life was nothing but a few more cycles of the moon. Eerily, a baby's cry was overheard in the hallway. "The circle of life," I thought. How often do we as physicians witness new beginnings and tragic endings? How often at the same time? The reality of medicine.

DEFEAT

One of the most important things I've learned during rotations is the immense amount of doubt that doctors feel, but do not express to patients. I have seen physicians enter a room and list the steps of the surgical procedure with confidence, then step out of the room and say, "I have no idea if I can remove that cancer." It is not deceiving. There is a finesse with which you speak to patients, especially if you are their last hope. Sometimes it is hope that you need to hear for yourself.

He had pancreatic cancer; which carries a frightening prognosis. He was already jaundiced with significant weight loss. Surgery to remove the cancer was his only chance at a cure. We were optimistic because the imaging studies informed us that the cancer had not "invaded" into surrounding structures, so we proceeded with surgery. If the cancer invades, you cannot continue. Studies have shown no benefit to survival plus you lengthen recovery time that they could have spent with their families.

In the OR, the residents knew immediately that it was non operable. They told me to take my hand and slide it under the vessel and feel that the pulse is diminished. This is because the cancer encapsulated it, restricting the blood flow. For them it was black and white. Invade or not invade? Proceed or do not proceed?

Dr. Jones was a passionate physician and he argued with the residents, "It has not invaded!!!" He had connected with the patient and their families before the procedure and told them that he would do his best. The residents understood his denial and stepped aside so that he could feel it for himself. When he did, the room was quiet. He never muttered the words, but instead stepped aside and let the residents close, without removing the cancer.

Dr. Jones sat in the corner of that operating room for the rest of the procedure, quietly defeated. This patient and their family would receive terrible news that afternoon. They would question his judgment, they would yell at him, scream, pull away from him. Their lives were forever changed. Not realizing that Dr. Jones had already taken that news with him and would carry that prognosis with him for the rest of his life as well.

JUST TELL ME

"The doctors won't give me a straight answer, I just want to know the truth. What's going on?"

The note had said that there were widespread metastases and palliative treatment had been initiated. A referral had been placed to hospice. Pancreatic cancer is unforgiving. Surely, this man had been told by at least one of the several doctors who had treated his cancer about his poor prognosis. Apparently not.

I hesitated. I was, of course, not the right person to tell him. He'd told me he had an eight-year-old son; this was a tragedy and I was a third-year medical student. This was way out of my league, I'd never done this before. I wanted to get out of there. I wanted to run away and not look back.

"I think your primary doctor will be by in a--"

"Just tell me what you know, kid. I'm tired of the games."

I hesitated. I might get in trouble, but I couldn't lie to him. So, I told him what I knew. I showed him CT his scan with a liver full of metastatic cancer. And then he started to cry. The magnitude of his pain overwhelmed me and I wanted so badly to get out of the room.

I sat in the chair next to his bed, trying desperately to come up with something comforting to say, but nothing came to mind.

He cried hard. My eyes were wet, too. I asked him if he wanted some privacy and he just mumbled, "nah." Maybe, I thought, he'd be more comfortable with company so that he wouldn't have to face the awful day alone. He was my only patient that day, so I stayed.

We didn't talk much: there wasn't much to say. Doctors came and went, nurses popped in. He cried intermittently, I just sat there. His oncologist confirmed the poor prognosis on the phone, saying he thought he'd explained it. Hours passed. I had felt trapped by the inability to help, suffocated by the lack of options. But by the end of the afternoon, I no longer had the urge to leave the room. I was right were I was supposed to be.

WANTED

An anatomy coloring book sent to work on after school. "Yes, Grandpa, neurosurgery sounds cool!" Months passed; the night before your visit, I scribbled frantically to make up progress I'd claimed on the phone. The next day, you lingered mercifully on the first, few, carefully colored pages, praising my work as I looked on anxiously: Is it what you wanted?

The white coat ceremony—we got here together—an old-school gentleman, you left when overcome with emotion. From the stage, I searched the crowd for your face. Is it what you wanted?

A phone call to discuss, with my newfound knowledge, the nuances of PSAs and PPVs. "Certainly," I reassured us both, "delaying the biopsy is fine—if it's what you wanted?"

When it wasn't fine, we talked again—about good times and proud moments. You wept (was it the hormones?). I didn't. Was it what you wanted?

Then you stopped answering, as I'd so often ignored you. "I don't want my grandson to see me like this," you told Mom. I was on Internal Medicine—I was being "dedicated"—seeing patients like yourself (but not you). Is it what you wanted?

They called, and I took notes on electrolytes and vent settings, as if it were just another board question. Sedate—and my multiple choice: to stay or to visit you. I stayed—is it what you wanted?

They called again, and this time, it was over. Refused treatment, this man so enamored of medicine? Ah, "I'm

treating myself," I learned you had said. At last, a
doctor—is it what you wanted?

Graduation approaches, only you won't be there, as I had
always imagined you would be. And seeing the road
before me—without you—I wonder, is it what you
wanted?

A SPECK OF SAND

My sister is in the hospital, water broken, 3 cm dilated, on epidural and oxytocin.

My sister is about to be a mother on Mother's Day.

I feel strongly about her baby. He will be the first born of my sister, the person that shares most of my childhood/adolescent/formative life. Just yesterday, my sister and I were playing House, experimenting with fried rice recipes, fighting over which channel to put the TV on. Just yesterday, we were climbing the mango tree in the backyard, going to church camp, flying to the States, and dancing at her wedding.

Ahmaud Arbery.

He would have been my age. I mourn for him. I mourn for his mother to whom he would have been saying "Happy Mother's Day" today. I mourn the truncation of the joy that his birth 26 years ago brought. I mourn the emptiness of the chair on which he would have been sitting, the space on the couch he would have been occupying. I mourn the confirmation of the fear into which he was born. I mourn his beauty, his humanity, the image of God in him.

I wonder about my sister's baby. I wonder how our relationship will be, how protective I'll be, how strict, how intense, how "cool." I wonder how much I'll love him. I wonder when I'll tell him about Ahmaud Arbery. I wonder how I'll tell him of the white cisheteropatriarchical society into which he is being born. I wonder how I'll teach him about his privilege, being born a male, being non-Black, being Christian, having a nurse mother, a respiratory therapist father, and a doctor uncle. I wonder if I will back off because he is not my child and I need to give him space.

I am a control freak; I try so hard to be in control. Yet, I am reminded every day that I am but a speck of sand in the grand scheme of the universe - a precious speck of sand - a speck of sand, nonetheless.

A speck of sand against a global pandemic.

A speck of sand against a crumbling democracy.

A speck of sand against anti-Black racism.

A speck of sand against the force of life that finds itself in the darkest and dreariest of days.

MINUTIAE

It took me nearly a year to realize why I was getting so little out of medical school. It wasn't that I was putting too little into it. Rather, it was that I was putting too much into the little things.

One more nerve. One more mechanism. One more factoid. What if these show up on the exam?

I was not learning to prepare myself to care for patients; I was learning to pass a test. Cram, regurgitate, forget; repeat.

The grandeur of life was always right in front of me, but I had made mine small. What if I don't pass this exam? Back to the lectures.

But somehow, life routinely brings me back to itself. Frequently, my little world is punctuated by invitations back to the big World.

Wait, do I need to know this for the exam? A patient erupts in tears before me as she shares that her sister has died.

I'm so stressed out by this upcoming presentation. My mom calls; her father passed this morning.

How high-yield is this for STEP1? My friend is thinking about harming himself; he refuses to seek care for his depression.

These lecture notes make no sense! Pandemic uproots the lives of millions.

Lately, I have had to reflect each day on the two most important lessons that this year has taught me: perspective and priority.

Perspective: What truly matters to me?

Priority: Am I living as if this were true?

Life mercifully reminds me, over and over again, of how often I fail to live in concordance with my perspectives and priorities, neither of which include laboring over minutiae. And it kindly – but firmly – invites me back to what matters most.

SECOND SELF

Do you ever feel like there are two of you?

When I started medical school, there was just one of me. The second one I sculpted to fit a need. Let's call her Second Self, or just Two for simplicity's sake.

Two was the studier. She was borne of lecture material and a Netter's Anatomical Atlas, suited to drawing connections in class, sitting at the kitchen table and absorbing information like a sponge. I tinkered with her here and there, made her more efficient at learning, capable of large intuitive leaps. She was a tool I created to survive the fire hose of information that is medical school.

But then she started to appear unsummoned, at inappropriate times, drawing connections I did not need. I really didn't need to think of a traffic jam on I95 as a deep vein thrombosis that embolized south like a clot through a blood vessel. But thanks anyway.

She became more easily activated. She stepped in because she thought she had to or else we would fail. She left the classroom and the kitchen table. She walked to class, not dancing in her head to music as I do, but thinking about today's schedule, reviewing the pharmacology from last night that she watched instead of Brooklyn 99. She noticed the leaves on the ground look like sphenoid bones of the skull.

She took more and more time from me, dressed in my clothes, wore my glasses, but only calculated beneath them. She doesn't paint; we don't have time for that in that shadow of a mountain of lecture material that awaits summitting. She became a shield I hide behind to

nurse my wounded ego when I do poorly on an exam.
She has no qualms about canceling plans, but is an
expert at avoiding them in the first place with five magic
words: "Sorry, I have to study."

She doesn't laugh that much. Her hands are filled with
chewed pencils that seem to litter the apartment of our
mind. She became the default. She turns off the alarm in
the morning. She sets it at night, calculating how much
time she needs and how early she wants to get to class. I
fight her here, battling for extra minutes of sleep. I push
the snooze button in the morning, knowing full well we'll
be late for class, just to spite her. To prove I'm still here,
buried beneath that avalanche of lecture material.
Sometimes battling for dominance; sometimes cowering
in shame. But still here.

PART TWO

TALES

OF

HUMOR

Laughter is the best medicine in the world.
— Milton Berle

Two things are infinite: the universe and human stupidity; and I'm not sure about the universe.
— Albert Einstein

There is nothing in the world so irresistibly contagious as laughter and good humor.
— Charles Dickens

BASICALLY A DOCTOR

The 4th and final year of medical school is a bizarre time. From the outsider's perspective, it's the culmination of 4. Whole. Years. You should basically be a doctor...right?

Well, between residency and graduation, interview season hits. In these interview-filled months, I went on 23 interviews, spent 100% of my mom's Southwest points she had collected over the last decade, gained 10% of my body weight at interview dinners, and lost 99% of all knowledge I ever gained in medical school.

You get off the plane. You struggle a bit to get your carry on suitcase out of the overhead bin (because MS4s never risk checking their suit) and do an awkward jog to the nearest airport bathroom. You try to shimmy off the Lululemon leggings that your sister (who went to graduate school for exactly 3 years to become a lawyer but makes more money than the rest of the doctors in your family combined) bought you while trying not to let your bare feet touch the nasty airport bathroom floor. You shake the wrinkles out of the familiar outfit that you wear to basically every pre-interview social and give it a sniff to make sure it smells okay, even though there's no alternative if it stinks. Spray some dry shampoo and switch out your Adidas for some Steve Madden. Stuff your stuff back into your bulging bag that contains supplies supposed to last at least 6 interviews. You jog to the passenger pick up area of the airport and see if Lyft or Uber is cheaper right now. Usually Lyft. You get in it.

"Are you just visiting for fun?"
"Oh, I'm actually in town for a job interview."
"Cool. What job?"
"I'm in medical school, and I am applying for residency."
"That's great. What kind of nurse will you be?"

You bring your carry on into the restaurant where the social is, and spend the next 2-3 hours chatting with other MS4s who also probably haven't been home in weeks. You get back to your hotel around 9 or 10 pm, struggle to fall asleep because you're scared you'll sleep through your alarm, and wake up just hours later, ready to take on interview day. Repeat.

Welcome to MS4. You're basically a doctor.

THE HUG

Lee and I had been on the trauma service for 26 hours at this point, and I was hungry, deliriously awake, and probably needed a breath mint. I was still coasting on the high hopes that I'd had at the start of our shift - I had seen my new resident around the hospital for weeks, and I was smitten by Lee's composure during emergencies, his magnetic presence, and unapologetic flair. I wasn't in love, I just desperately wanted to be his friend. When I saw that we had been paired up for a full 24-hour shift, it felt too good to be true.

Lee was tougher than I expected him to be. He casually expressed disappointment with my physical exam, and he sent me back to try again. He pushed me to present to him without my eyes glued on my notes. He said I should carry around plenty of wound dressing supplies, just in case. Even though we didn't have grades, I wanted to impress him. Early in our shift, he had promised to discuss career tips, but the night picked up quick so we never got the chance. Sometimes he was so deep in thought, preoccupied by the demands of our service, that he didn't hear my questions.

Slowly the night turned to morning, and we were on our way to wake up a few patients before rounds. Buoyed by our 5 AM bout of wired laughter over something that wouldn't be so funny any other time of day, I was feeling hopeful that Lee had come to like me too. My suspicion was confirmed when Lee reached one arm over towards me. I was ecstatic. Naturally, I reciprocated the hug. As I wrapped my hands around his shoulders, time slowed down. Had the scene been a cartoon, the soundtrack would have abruptly changed to screeching brakes - I realized Lee's outstretched arm had been reaching for the elevator button on the wall behind me. It seemed that I had misread the situation. I untangled myself, too tired to be sheepish. Lee was too focused on rounding to show discomfort or pity with my unsolicited affection. Offhandedly he said he'd give me a hug later, a promise I figured he'd forget like the others, and off we went to complete our morning tasks.

Incredibly, when our 24 (which was really a 27 but who's counting?) wrapped up and we walked down to the cafeteria, after Lee paid for my breakfast, and it seemed like we were about to part ways, Lee initiated an embrace. He remembered. I felt so special. A few weeks later I learned our budding friendship didn't quite result in a favorable evaluation of my clinical skills... but I'll never forget that hug.

A TRICKY TREMOR

I conducted a cursory chart review of the patient I would be seeing for afternoon neurology clinic. I saw a referral note stating that the patient had a tremor and was being referred for suspected Parkinson's disease.

"Oh I know this!" I thought to myself, going over the TRAPS mnemonic that describes common symptoms associated with Parkinson's. "Tremor...rigidity..."

I jotted down what physical exam findings to take extra note of before entering the room. I was greeted by an elderly woman and her daughter, both of whom were very courteous. I breathed a sigh of relief that they were not disappointed to be seeing a medical student first.

"Hm... well you're not really rigid," I said, as I extended and flexed the patient's arm. "And your tremor looks like it is not at rest. My assessment is that this is probably not Parkinson's disease."

I quickly organized my data before presenting my findings to the attending.

"So, you think this is essential tremor - not Parkinson's disease? Let's see if you were right."

I watched as my attending adeptly performed the same maneuvers that I had done to assess the patient's neurologic status. Except when he performed them, he came to a much different conclusion.

"You see this, what I'm doing? She has a tiny bit of resistance here that is consistent with cogwheel rigidity," he stated, as he flexed and extended the patient's arm just as I had.

One strike.

"And this tremor? It actually is at rest- she fooled you by focusing on the tremor to calm it down."

Two strikes.

"It appears to me that you have classic symptoms of Parkinson's disease," the attending stated calmly to the patient.

Three strikes. I had completely miscalculated my clinical interpretation of a disease that I had only studied in books.

"Don't worry," the attending said to me when I expressed my combination of embarrassment and sadness. "This is what training is for!"

"SHOE"LD NOT HAVE DONE THAT

After much deliberation, I decided to wear my black kitten heels to my first shadowing experience to boost my humble height of 4'11 to 5'0 flat. My worn-down Adidas sneakers simply do not scream "student doctor," despite their comfort to my feet. Every medical student wants to dress up to the nines when they first enter the hospital as a student doctor. After all, if we were to be in cool places like the ER, we might as well look great for the occasion – right?

With my school's encouragement, I decided on a fancy outfit for my first day as a student doctor. I felt confident in my kitten heels; after all, good heels take you to good places. Except when nature decides to rain on your parade. After an hour of downpour, the hospital grounds were soft as melted marshmallow. I struggled to walk; kitten heels digging into mush with every step.

When the time came for us to walk with our attending and ride an elevator, I rushed in first in fear of being left behind. Suddenly, I felt a strong tug on my foot, looked down, and in horror, found my right kitten heel stuck in the elevator gap. At that point, I'd rather run around the halls wearing nothing but a flimsy hospital gown than be in front of everybody struggling to free my poor kitten heels.

My beloved heels turned to be my shoes of shame. Everywhere I went, doctors looked down on my shoes with disapproving eyes. Everyone in the ER wore sneakers. I tried hiding my shoes by standing at the back of the group. Of course, the loud "clack clack" of my shoes did not help my attempt at hiding at all. Finally, my attending scolded me in front of the ER, saying "I like your shoes, they look gorgeous on you. But there is no way you'll enter my ER with those shoes again." I apologized and promised to never do it again. Deep down, I had a strong urge to take my shoes off and run bare-footed out of the ER, find a closet, and drown in my embarrassment.

I definitely learned a good lesson that day. I found myself investing in mud and elevator gap resistant, hospital friendly sneakers ever since. My kitten heels never saw the light of day again. They sit at the back of my closet because sometimes I stare at them and remember that day. My only consolation was that hey, at least I looked good on my first day!

LIFE OF A THIRD YEAR

For whatever reason, it was notoriously difficult to get "honors" evaluations on my school's pediatrics rotation. One day, I set out to change that.

I was assigned to work in the afternoon clinic with one of the senior residents. The resident seemed very nice and friendly (always a plus when you are looking for a good evaluation). Being towards the back end of the rotation, I was finally gaining some confidence in my abilities. I volunteered to see as many patients as I could, noticing that it was a particularly packed schedule that day.

I saw the patients as quickly and thoroughly as possible.

I gave the most succinct presentation I could after each visit, highlighting the most salient points gracefully

I exuded genuine excitement about the field of pediatrics.

I formed connections with the kids and the parents.

I even helped to translate a foreign language for the resident in a room where all of the children were infested with lice and bouncing off the walls at a million miles an hour.

At the end of the exhausting day, the resident thanked me for my work calling me "one of the best medical students to work with."

At this point, I could already taste an evaluation with all "honors," the greatest reward any third year medical student can hope to receive for their efforts.

I handed over my evaluation card, politely asking to have it filled out. And for the first time in a long time, I actually did so with confidence.

As I happily snuck out of the room, I quickly scanned over the evaluation.

Final Grade: "Pass," not "Honors."

Surely, I had misread it.

Unfortunately, not.

Instead, it was just another day as a third-year medical student.

MASKED SUPERHEROES

During the early days of the COVID-19 pandemic, I prepared to interview my patient. We were both cognizant of the risks of the virus, and we agreed that surgical masks would be the order of the day for both of us.

In my fledgling medical career, I have noted that I could make most patients chuckle and some genuinely laugh during an interview. My dry sense of humor was particularly effective if I saw the patient's facial expressions and he or she saw mine. That day in mid-March though, the technique that came naturally to me, wasn't working. My usual rapport with the patient was lacking and I could tell that the mask had everything to do with it. With the patient unable to see my facial expression and I unable to make out his, my dry sense of humor fell short. Building a relationship was not as easy as it used to be.

If that wasn't enough, my mask also embarrassed me with my attending physician! "Here to pick up the patient for x-ray huh?" I had called out to the hazel-eyed, thin, young-looking woman who was walking towards the patient's room. "Steven, I am Dr. Grey," the current *Doctor of the Year*, calmly replied.

Outside of the med school setting, it was no different. I could have been faulted for being lazy at times and running to the supermarket in my private scrubs. But these are different days. My usual quiet confidence of being a medical student on a worthwhile pursuit was replaced by uneasiness at people who shot me suspicious glances over their masked noses and mouths, worried if I was a greater harbinger of infection than anyone else there.

Regardless, we continue to tread on uncharted grounds into the unknown. As our practices of social distancing and wearing masks become the new normal, for me the stresses of today are relieved by the laughs I picture when I one day tell my grandchildren how the heroes of COVID-19 looked like astronauts, geared up in spacesuits, and gravitating 6 feet apart.

Not all superheroes wear capes, some wear masks.

SCABIES POSITIVE

As you quickly find out being a 3rd year medical student, sometimes the only things you can offer the team are faxing for outside records, calling Walgreens pharmacy for a patient's med list, or bringing back leftovers from lunch conference. When you are given a task – any task – you want to do it well.

On my first day of Internal Medicine wards, our new admit was assigned to me. "Finally!" I thought, "My time to shine." I grabbed my MS3 partner, Albert, and flew down to the ER.

Our patient was a tall, scraggly, elderly gentleman with scant gray hair. "Hello Mr. H!" I exclaimed, quickly noticing some red flags as he began itching the scabs on his arms and shared, "I'm livin' on the streets." Eagar to get started, I was ready to examine his scabs when Albert whispered, "Wear gloves!" Right, of course!

"Thank you, Mr. H, "I said, as I finished and tossed my gloves.

"Wait!" yelled Mr. H. "Can you put my ID away?"

"Sure!" Not wanting to be impolite, I thought, "Yeah, I don't need gloves to touch an ID card, right?"

"Here, it's in my street clothes," said Mr. H as he dumped a pile of soiled clothing onto my chest. I froze...then took a deep breath and put away his belongings. Having successfully obtained an MS3-quality H&P, Albert and I marched back to the workroom, chins up high and hands on our hips as we grinned, "We got the history!"

Our senior resident rolled his chair away from the door faster than you can say "99." Eyes wide, he asked, "Are you guys itchy? Derm just dropped their note on that guy in the

ER...scabies." He began explaining, "You'll need to get your white coats cleaned, you have to get this special cream for treatment..." But all I could think was, "Scabies??? GAME OVER ON THE FIRST DAY! Maybe I'm not cut out for this..." My mind was racing in panic. Before I could even finish thinking about how many showers I wanted to take, Dermatology suddenly called.

"Howdy, it's Derm! I'll go see that guy Mr. H."

"You didn't see him yet? Your note said he has scabies..." questioned our senior resident.

"No no, I just pre-wrote the note, haven't seen him yet," she replied.

Shortly after she called back, "Just saw Mr. H. It's not scabies, thanks!" We all exhaled in relief. As our senior resident lectured me that I should've called him, should've worn gloves, etc....all I thought was "Great. Now there's no way I'm getting Honors!"

TAKING ONE FOR THE TEAM

Pediatric patients are some of the most complex for several reasons. For one, they often cannot explain their symptoms well and present entirely differently than adults. Secondly, they are known to be fraught with jokes and unpredictability, making each day a unique experience. For these reasons, unorthodox approaches are mastered by pediatricians when treating children. I experienced firsthand the importance of these tactics early in my pediatrics rotation with my 7-year-old patient, Zoey.

Zoey had a headache and nausea for over six days. As part of our work up, blood tests were needed and an IV had to be inserted. When I told her and her parents this, she adamantly rejected the idea of a needle being put in her arm, let alone it staying for a few hours. As I explained to her that they are very common and she may only feel a pinch, I ran into a dilemma. I fell into a trap that does not happen very much in other fields besides pediatrics.

I was asked to prove it.

Though truthfully afraid of needles myself, I was desperate to be an asset for Zoey and my team. And as I learned early on, an unhappy child on the floor makes for an unhappy team. So, I did what any good team member would do and agreed to appease Zoey. As the nurse placed an IV in my arm in front of her, I was battling to not let my true emotions surface. After what had to be the hardest examination I had taken in school, my fabricated blunting of pain passed Zoey's test, and she finally became comfortable with getting one herself. By agreeing to her unusual request, in fifteen minutes there was an IV in both Zoey and me, a small fee to pay for her trust. As I left the hospital that day and came home to my roommate asking what happened to me while pointing to the Spiderman Band-Aid on my arm, I shrugged it off and thought to myself, "just another day."

A GULLIBLE GULP

We were finishing up Teaching Rounds, a time where we as students could play attending and take our classmates through the wards to meet and treat our most interesting patients. Moving on to the next activity, I huffed and puffed up 10 flights of stairs, making it first to the top. Being the nice guy that I am, I proceeded to hold the door open for the rest of the crew.

"You're welcome!" I smiled as I followed the last student into the breakroom, where my friend was handing out much needed water cups to the whole group. "Yo, Gabe! So are we taking a water break or what?" I asked as he passed me the last cup. "Yup!" he laughed.

"Perfect, I'm parched!" I thought to myself, staying behind to gulp down 3 cups. I marched my way over to the conference room only to find all of my classmates sitting in a circle, filled water cups on their desks, and my attending demonstrating a proper palpation of his thyroid for the class. Janelle chuckled, "Where's your water cup!? Did you think we were just taking a water break or something? We're practicing thyroid exams dude!"

I froze in front of the laughter-struck class. "That's exactly what I was thinking..." As I handed my attending my empty water cup and palpated his dry neck as he gulped air, I knew my gullible gulp would be my unintentional claim to fame for the rest of medical school.

AN UNEXPECTED GIFT

I was on my two-week urology rotation, watching the intern prep our patient for kidney stone removal surgery. It was the middle of my surgery block, and my mood was at an all-time low. After the anesthesiologist confirmed that the patient was unconscious, I helped the intern position the patient properly, on his back with his feet propped up on stirrups and buttocks pushed to the edge of the table. I stood back as the intern carefully cleaned the area around his genitals and buttocks with chlorhexidine antiseptic. He was crouching down, working his way around the anus, when he turned and looked at me, eyes wide behind his goggles.

"Oh no, look what we've got here..."

We both watched with disbelief as an enormous turd—ahem, stool—started creeping out of our patient's anus. It was the closest, most unobstructed view I had ever had to an adult-sized bowel movement in action. It seemed to move in slow motion.

"This guy did not follow the pre-op guidelines."

I watched in awe as the intern put on a new set of gloves, and, when the log seemed to be finally tapering to an end, helped pinch it off into a trash can. He changed his gloves again and immediately got back to work re-cleaning the area. This was a truly stellar intern.

Three minutes had not passed before the scene started to repeat itself.

"No, no, no, no..."

We stood back and watched again as another turd announced itself. The intern sighed. This was not his morning. I tried and failed to stifle my laughter as he once again held up the trash can, pinched off the log, and began one more time to sterilize the area.

Thankfully, there was no lucky number three. But because of some operating room formality that forbids trash bags from being removed from a room once a procedure has officially started, the entire team – the anesthesiologist, attending, senior resident, intern, circulating nurse, surgical tech, and I – spent the next two hours intermittently holding our breath. And I spent the next week crying with laughter each time I recounted the story to another unwitting audience.

That patient will never know how much joy he brought me.

EYES N' NOSE

It's the morning of the first day of my first 3rd year clerkship, Surgical Oncology. My kind intern, Barbara, quickly ran me through how to pre-round on patients. She gave me many helpful tips – "Always ask about their pain level, whether they've peed, if they've passed gas, if they've been nauseous or vomited, and if they've been able to walk. Gather their vital signs before rounds and keep your presentation short - no more than 2 minutes." I appreciated and took her advice seriously. Rushing out the door to see her own patients, Barbara stops to add, "Oh, and always check their eyes and nose – they [senior residents and attendings] will always want to know about their eyes and nose."

Every morning before dawn, I reported to the hospital to pre-round on my assigned patients. I reviewed any overnight nursing notes, jotted down their vital signs, and went to their bedside to gather histories and physical exams. I asked all of the questions that Barbara advised, checked their surgical wound(s), and made sure to check their eyes and nose. Were their sclerae icteric? Conjunctiva injected? Were their pupils dilated? Or equal, round, and reactive? Was there nasal flaring? Swollen turbinates? Sinus tenderness?

We are taught that, especially early in our medical training, there is no such thing as being "too thorough." Even so, examining the eyes and nose of patients who'd just had an abdominal tumor removed didn't quite make sense to me (particularly considering that I was waking them at 5am!), but I did it anyway because, well, I was instructed to do so. As we are reminded over and over again, presentations are a medical student's "time to shine." So, talking as fast as I could, sweat under my arms, I confidently delivered brief presentations of my patients each morning. I made sure they included pain level, pee/poo/fart data; vital signs; whether their incision was clean, dry, and intact; whether their pupils were equal, round, and reactive; and whether their nose was atraumatic or nontender..."

During the fourth and final week of this rotation, I was running to keep up with the residents on rounds, as usual, when Barbara turned around and asked me, "Could you do me a favor and write down this patient's eyes and nose?"

"Sorry?" I said, confused. "What do you mean 'write down her eyes and nose'?"

She shot back, "Her I's and O's!... her ins and outs!"

ONCE UPON A RECTAL

My first real patient encounter ended in the most unconventional way. Everything was going fine. I introduced myself to my preceptor. We talked, discussed real life practice, discussed med school and residency. I even got to observe her patient encounters that day. I'll never forget it. Wearing your white coat in front of a real patient not a paid actor – this was the dream!

The day goes on and we see her last patient. She tells her nurse to glove me and proceeds to put lubricant jelly and instructs, "now remember, slide, insert, and twist."

Oh, did I mention my preceptor was a colorectal surgeon?

Well there it happened, I performed my first rectal exam on my first day. What a rush.

This was a skill we were set to learn in the next two months, and I had done it (and done it well might I add). That was definitely going to be my biggest boast at our next social gathering.

Fast forward two months later, and it was time to learn and do the feared rectal exam in class. "what if my nails are too long?" "What if I hurt the patient?" All my classmates were worried and caught off guard and I proceeded to show them the "slide, insert, and twist" method. And sure enough, they all succeeded.

I'll never forget one classmate exclaiming "I'll always remember you as the girl who taught me how to perform a rectal exam."

There we have it folks, my biggest claim to fame!

A STOOL NOT FOR SITTING

I smoothed down my white coat and adjusted my stethoscope. I straightened my name tag and pushed my shoulders back. I mentally ran through the checklist of interview skills that had been provided in the student guide: "Introduce yourself to everyone in the room, find out what your patient prefers to be called, say something to put the patient at ease." I squeezed some hand sanitizer onto my clammy hands and walked into the hospital room, hoping my legs were not visibly shaking.

It was my first day in the hospital. My first experience medically interviewing a patient. It was a BIG day. My preceptor stood off to the side, watching and waiting to intervene at any point. With a huge smile across my face, I walked over to the patient to shake her hand and introduce myself. She smiled back. So far, so good.

My brain scrambled through the checklist again, remembering an important point - positioning is key. The student guide had emphasized sitting down, even grabbing a chair from elsewhere if need be, because a good interview required being at eye level with the patient. I was not about to mess that up. I scanned the room for a chair while still trying to maintain eye contact with the patient. Lo and behold, there was a chair right next to her bed, already perfectly placed for me. My heart started to beat a little more slowly; everything seemed to be working out. I settled into the chair and pulled out my notepad, ready to commence what felt like the most important interview of my life.

Then I heard my preceptor clear his throat. I turned to look at him, pure shock in his eyes. "Margot," he whispered as he gestured to my perfectly placed chair, "that's a commode."

EXTREME EMPATHY

I opened my eyes to a doctor standing over me, a nurse wheeling in a wheelchair, and a young boy staring at me with large, frightened eyes. I thought to myself, "Oh no, did this really just happen?"

"Everything's okay. You passed out and hit your head against the wall," the doctor explained. Yep, it happened.

I quickly stood up, profusely apologized to the boy, and tried to dart out of the room. But as if I wasn't embarrassed enough, they sat me down in the wheelchair and wheeled me into the exam room next door. And that is how I found myself admitted to the pediatric emergency room as an MS1 student.

But let me start from the beginning. I've always fainted easily from the presence of pain. It doesn't take much - a game of red rover, slamming a finger in the car door, bumping an elbow on the wall, period cramps. It wasn't until I fainted in a Ralph Lauren retail store in middle school that I finally saw a doctor. The diagnosis: a low heart rate and vasovagal syncope. I worked hard to prevent further episodes, but that wasn't the case on that fateful day in the pediatric ER.

"A 7-year-old boy presents today with a possible concussion due to a mountain biking accident." I followed the attending into the room and observed him perform a history and physical. The boy had a large hematoma in the middle of his forehead. The attending started pressing on the bump; pressing so hard that the boy began writhing and wincing in pain. As I watched, the boy's pain hit me right in the gut. I started to feel cold sweats and chills. "Don't give in," I told myself. I reached for the stool under the computer and took a seat.

As I sat down, a wave of black came over me, causing me to fall off the stool and hit my head against the wall.

As I sat in the ER bed, the heat of embarrassment burned through my cheeks. I saw the attending return to the boy's exam room with a plethora of stickers. The nurses and doctors encouraged me that it happens to the best, but the shame stung.

When I was finally discharged and returned home, I looked in the mirror to find I now had a hematoma in the middle of my forehead. I had felt the boy's pain so intensely that I passed out and ended up with the same bump. I congratulated myself on the ability to have extreme empathy. Or at least, that's what I told myself to get through the embarrassment. Now, all I have to show for my extreme empathy are two scars and a $400 bill to the ER.

A NEW LEVEL OF COMMITMENT

It's the first week of my psychiatry clerkship. I've been placed for the month on an involuntary long-term inpatient ward. Here I am, hanging around on the floor, trying to look busy and impressive. It's a new rotation, and the 9AM psych rotation start-time has me feeling energetic and ready to snag that Honors. Nothing can stop me.

An older gentleman, maybe in his mid-70s, approaches me, and begins shouting in a foreign language. He sounds like he's trying desperately to communicate something. One of the residents, also new on the floor, and no doubt seeing me glancing around sideways for help, walks over and tries to talk to the man, but to no avail. "Do you speak Spanish?" he asks. "I do," I reply, "but I don't think this is Spanish." It sounds Eastern European. Maybe Russian?

The man is becoming more agitated. He walks over to the locked door leading out of the ward and rattles the handle. Then he starts banging on the door and walls. The other patients come over to watch. We beckon the man back to his room, and he follows, marching like he's ready to go to war. We call his nurse over, who tells us Leon has been manic, refusing medications, and making repeated escape attempts over the past week. He only speaks Polish and is frustrated that no one seems to understand that he is not meant to be here at all.

The resident is contemplating an injection cocktail, though none of us is too eager, as Leon doesn't exactly seem like a danger to himself or anyone else. However, we still need to treat him. Spying his uneaten breakfast sitting on a table, I come up with the idea to mix Leon's Depakote into his yogurt. The resident agrees to try, and the nurse quietly adds it to the food while Leon isn't looking.

I sit down at the table and offer him the food. He won't eat it. So I grab a new, unopened container of yogurt, pull out Google translate, search "I eat, you eat" in Polish, and dig in. It's working! Leon follows my lead and starts to eat his too. We sit in companionable silence for a few minutes, me marveling at my own brilliance and congratulating myself on the amazing impression I must surely have made on this resident. Would he tell this story to his colleagues? "You'll never believe what my med student came up with... isn't that genius!"

Suddenly however, Leon notices everyone watching, and realizes a trick has been played. He points at my cup, gesturing to switch. I hang my head and accept defeat. Some things aren't worth the grade bump.

HEALING HANDS

"Rooney, I need you for something."
"Of course, sir," I almost instinctively replied, eager to prove my worth to my attending.
"Remind me again, what is it you're interested in pursuing for residency?"
"Well, sir, radiology, but I'm still keeping my options open."
"Oh good, I want you to look at the CT scan that just came in for room 6. Tell me what you see."

While logging into the EMR system, I quickly glanced at the triage board and read "constipation" under the chief complaint.

"So, what do you see, Rooney"
"Well, sir, a lot of stool," I proudly exclaimed while simultaneously tracing the large bowel loops with my fingers.
"Exactly, good job. Now, how do you want to fix it?"
Now feeling slightly apprehensive, I unconfidently replied, "A laxative?"

"No Rooney," my preceptor replied grinning, "with your healing hands," as chuckling now began to erupt from surrounding staff.

And that's how I managed to perform my first manual fecal disimpaction. I'm not convinced showing too much enthusiasm or mentioning my interest in pursuing radiology may have been in my best interest but I suppose it did help with honoring the rotation.

ARE YOU A DOCTA?

It was my first clerkship of MS3, rotating in a busy county psych emergency department. We had a new admit: a schizophrenic patient with suicidal ideation. She was having auditory hallucinations and was quite paranoid. I introduced myself and began to gather a history. We were in the hall, waiting for the admit staff to figure out a room for her.

A younger female patient, also psychotic, was strolling down the hall. She jumped in mid-sentence; "HI!"

"Oh, um hi," I quickly replied. Back to my patient, "So, tell me mor—"

"How you doing?" she drawled, looking me up and down.

Suddenly having a Joey Tribbiani – Friends flashback, I stuttered back, "Uhh, I'm good, thanks!" I tried to turn back to my patient. "Tell me more about these voi--"

"So...so are you a docta?" she asked, in a voice significantly more flirtatious than I had heard since I started STEP studying.

Despite it being a nice change at 3pm in the windowless ED, I quickly set her straight.

"Nope!"

My schizophrenic patient, who had logically assumed I was at least somewhat qualified, bolted to attention. Her eyes widened. "WHAT???"

Ah well.

WORLD CUP FEVER

Jumping out of the car from the hospital parking lot, I scrambled a dress shirt over my Brazil jersey, throwing a 5-second Windsor knot as seen on YouTube, as we ran toward the double doors. Like any good pair of med students would, my colleague and I arrived to an empty workroom 3 hours before rounds. Settling in to my computer, my fingers typed at the speed of light, logging me into...ESPN!

World Cup Soccer arrives only once every 4 years, and nothing was going to get in the way of Kevin and I enjoying every moment. I adjusted my dual monitors for maximum efficiency, one game on the left screen, the other on the right. Feet crossed on the desk, hands behind our heads, and hearing "Gooooool de Lionel Messi!!!" was more our type of Morning Report.

Evidently, we weren't the only ones in the hospital who caught World Cup Fever. In the middle of rounds, the janitor's voice, "That's a penalty!" echoed through the hallways as he pretended to work by mopping the same tile for the thousandth time. Before I could yell, "red card!" the janitor had his garbage can on the ground as a goal, rolling a gown into a ball. Reenacting the scene, he put on an Academy Award-winning performance as he dribbled through our team huddle to take a dive to the floor that Neymar himself would be proud of.

Nor was our attending immune to the contagious spirit filling the hospital. Dr. Lindsey guided us to the bedside of Mr. T once again. Though this 91-year-old man hadn't spoken a full sentence all week, Dr. Lindsey was convinced he was an oracle for the World Cup. His prophecy proved impeccable for 10 games out of 10 so far, and we expected no less for the World Cup Final.

"So Mr. T who's gonna win today's big game – France or Croatia???" Slurping his yogurt as the speech pathologist fed him, he slurred, "Crrroayysha." My heart skipped a beat, taking his word for the holy truth. We would learn two things later that day: 1. Mr. T's final prophecy couldn't have been further from the truth. 2. His MOCA score for dementia returned as 1 point out of 30.

As we celebrated France's win over a couple plates of mystery meat at noon conference, we were overjoyed when the 20 attendings in the room asked us to throw on highlights of the game on the projector. We happily obliged. Would this be a good time to ask for feedback?

THANK YOU STEP ONE

I stumble out the door. My body is wiped, my brain so numb it hurts.

It had been rainy and gray when I entered that sad, solitary structure at 7:30 AM. It's 2:43 PM now and my rain jacket is shoved on top of a bag of uneaten snacks and emergency supplies (contact solution, Band-Aids for possible paper cuts, Advil, hand sanitizer, a face mask). As I zigzag my way through the parking lot, drunk on a cocktail of elation, defeat, and relief, I am blinded by the warm May light. My skin drinks in the UV and I can almost feel my body synthesizing the vitamin D it has been deprived of since early April. A loiterer stares at me with a sneer. I'm not sure if he's mocking my gait (it's not a cerebellar problem) or if he's thinking to himself that I'm the palest Californian he's ever seen.

I'm close to my destination now, but I'm not quite ready to leave it all behind yet, not without some last words. So I start composing a letter in my head that goes something like this...

Thank you Step One, my one constant these past COVID weeks. Though our relationship
    was turbulent at times, you have been a loyal friend despite the indecisiveness you
    displayed towards the end (I had to reschedule four times because of you!). I assure
    you, everything is forgiven. But I think you and I agree that it's time we both move on,
    move on to real people and living things. I will always be grateful for all you have
    taught me, and don't worry, I have a feeling we'll see each other around soon. I hear
    there's something called Step Two.

I sign my name and carefully tuck the letter into an imaginary envelope before turning back for a last look at the place where this chapter is coming to a close. It's really too bad it has to be in a cracked asphalt patch across from the flashing lights of the Hustler Casino. Though not as picturesque as I had hoped, it's over. I'm not sure I passed, but I still can't help but feel I've come out on the winning end. Like the end to any inspirational sports movie, the metaphorical fans are cheering, my teammates are crushed in a pile of bodies, and the victory song plays as I drive home, dreaming about the many dark, damp corners in my closet that will soon become First Aid's final resting place.

THE COUPLES MATCH CONUNDRUM

Ding dong. "That's my package!" David and I yelled in sync. We had both been buying clothes on Amazon to get ready for the couples match season. As a Family Medicine applicant, I could already feel the rays of sunlight toasting my skin on the beach at my top program. But I couldn't get too excited – David's Derm dreams might lead us to the middle of nowhere, keeping us far away from toasty skin. I opened the package to find my bikini, right next to David's new winter coat. After throwing an approving glance at his new purchase, David rushed out the door yelling, "Babe you won't be needing that bikini if we match in Podunk!"

Podunk?! Where in the world is Podunk?! I consulted Dr. Google: "Top ten things to do in Podunk." All sites unanimously arrived at the same conclusion: baking potatoes and cow tipping. Fine, but maybe it's by the beach? "Weather in Podunk" click. "Negative infinite Celcius." Well, I thought to myself, "the only toasting I am going to do is with the potatoes."

We soon landed in Podunk for interview day, snow seeping through my flip flops. The resident hosting us called me, "Hi! So what brings you out to Podunk?" I excitedly shared, "I have family in the area!" I refrained from saying that this 'family' was my 4th cousin Larry, twice removed, that lives 3 states over.

In Podunk or not, we are in this together, I reminded myself. I had to look on the bright side, we will finally be earning our first paychecks! While our non-medical school friends have a house and kids, we are sharing a 1996 Chrysler Sebring convertible, convincing ourselves that opening the roof makes up for the wonky gears. As much as my parents want us to match at the community hospital across the street from their house, of course, there's no Derm program for David in sight.

Such is life with the couples match, but all in all, we are truly excited for whatever the future has in store. I am happy to trade in my bikini for a winter coat if it means I'm with you.

IS THERE
A DOCTOR IN THE HOUSE?

As a medical student, you find potential patients everywhere. Whether you're on an airplane or on a romantic dinner date, we've all heard those famous words, "Is there a doctor in the house?!" Here are some of my favorite "patient" encounters.

The best friend curbside. I was playing ball with my boys – that's right FIFA on the PlayStation – when my buddy drops the question, "So listen man, you're a doctor right? I need some advice about my knee, it's been killing me! I landed weird after jumping during soccer the other week, and now it's been aching ever since."

Assessment and Plan: 27-year-old man, clearly delusional as he thinks I'm a doctor, presents to FIFA night complaining of right knee pain. Obviously, he should rest, ice it, use compression, and elevate the leg, right?

He continued, "So I went to my primary care doc and he told me to rest, ice it, use compression, and elevate the leg! Isn't that the dumbest thing you ever heard?" Uh oh, I couldn't blow my cover, "Yeah totally ... maybe you should get that checked out!"

The jacuzzi. Practicing your interviewing questions for your STEP 2 Clinical Skills exam can be a drag, so my roommate and I decided to hop in the jacuzzi of our apartment complex: cold iced teas in one hand, First Aid books in the other. The jacuzzi was packed, but we stayed in our own world practicing cases. Next thing you know, the gentleman next to us asked for a consult! "Hey bud! Luckily I don't have the discharge when I pee like you're buddy over here, but I got this mole on my back. You mind taking a look at it for me?" Well, no better way to practice than the real deal!

The rugby game. Beaming with humanism, my buddy and I volunteered to be sports medics on the sidelines of a youth rugby game. We figured there would be an official team of sports physicians, and we were happy to designate ourselves as the Band-Aid service. Arriving at the venue, I told my friend nervously, "Dude...I think we might be the only 'medics' here." Five minutes into the game, the whistle blows, "We need a medic!" Yikes. We both run onto the field, praying that the kid is fine. "Hey are you okay?" I ask the kid, who was lying on the ground, staring absently at the sky. He smiles, "Yup! Just feels good to lay down here." Phew! The game resumes.

A half hour later, a gentleman runs up to us. "My wife isn't feeling too well, can you take a look?" We find the wife, who fortunately looks fresh as a daisy. "I'm just a little tired, I haven't eaten all morning," she says. "She usually feels better with a mint," the husband chimes in. After a full history and advising her to hydrate and eat lunch, we are ready to write the prescription. "Got any mints?" I whisper to my buddy. With that, we give out our first prescription – a spearmint Altoid!

SONG AND DANCE

Everything in medical school seems to start out similarly to learning a song and dance. You walk into the standardized patient's (SP) room for the first time and out of your mouth jumps, "H-Hello, I'm a med student."

The SP (a word of a song that those long-gone MS3's have thrown around) gives you The Look. You know the one. The one that adults used to give you when you'd tell them that one day, you'll be elected Ruler of the World, with the wisp of a smile at the corner of their lips and those little amused wrinkles around their eyes. They say it's okay, lots of students are nervous on their first time. Would you like to try again? Oh yeah, and please wash your hands first this time.

Those are the first steps to your dance. The first words to your song.

I memorized that song and dance, because it'll make me a doctor. "Hello, my name is student. I go to school. I'm working with your doctor today and he asked me to come in and do an exam of some sort on you. Is that alright with you? Great. Now first, let me lower your exam table to 30 degrees and pull out the- Wait, wait, I forgot to wash my hands! Please don't dock my points."

When I went to volunteer at a free clinic for the first time, I was ready. It's the same song and dance. The only difference? I'm not getting graded. Yes!

I entered and there she was. My first REAL patient. No SP's. I sang the first words of the song: Hello, how are you? I did the first step of the dance: I washed my hands.

And then, she changed the tune.

Before I could say a word, she was already speaking. She had come in for a medication refill, pain in her shoulder, and flecks in her urine. She was already dumping bottle after bottle of medication from her purse. This one's a water pill and this one's a heart pill and these are all diabetes pills and she isn't sure what this one's for, but it tastes weird and –

She adds words to the song, ones I don't know yet. I recognize medication names, but don't know what they mean. She also has an EKG, can I read it for her? That's a dance step that I know for sure I missed on that last exam. And this one has even more lines and artifacts. And did someone put her leads on backwards?

After a million years, she goes quiet. Then, she throws back her head and laughs. I stare at her, still stuck on what in the world furosemide was. Was this another part of the song that I never learned?

"Oh, don't look so shocked! You look like you need the doctor more than I do right now!"

WHAT'S IN A NAME

English is already weird enough, but sometimes the language of medicine is outright bizarre. Don't get me wrong, once in a while we name medical terms in a perfectly sensible way. For example, congestive heart failure tells you a lot about the condition simply through the name. Ancylostoma duodenale, if you look at the Greek roots, means "hook mouth in the duodenum," and this, too, makes a good bit of sense if you consider the morphology of this little worm and its preferred abode.

Nevertheless, I have spent much of my first year in medical school in a state of outright confusion over how certain names were engrained into our culture and have withstood the test of time.

Malassezia furfur. With all due respect to Mr. Malassez, endowing this fungus with your surname has resulted in many sleepless study nights reviewing my microbiology Anki cards, hoping to find a logical mnemonic to memorize the name – to no avail! And, indeed, each time I encountered a disease or even a body part named after someone, I asked myself, "Why on Earth did this person want their memory to be preserved in such a way?" I can understand leaving your mark in history with your name on a building, a statue in a park, or even your face engraved in a mountain! But, naming a germ after yourself? That is some next-level thinking.

Francisella tularensis. Named after Dr. Edward Francis and the discovery of the bacterium in squirrels of Tulare County, California. Not only did this man once again endow a microbe with his name, but he also associated the residents of Tulare with this rather terrifying pathogen and potential biochemical weapon.

There are, fortunately, times when a poorly named medical term does not bring anguish but rather a laugh: the pouch of Douglas (not a useful name), also known as the recto-uterine pouch (a useful name). It will never cease to make me giggle that the extension of the peritoneal cavity between the rectum and the uterus is named after a man, Mr. James Douglas. Ironically, out of all the bits of anatomy that I have studied and then forgotten, the pouch of Douglas is actually a humorous term that will forever be engrained in memory. Thanks for the laugh, Mr. Douglas!

If you want a final challenge, riddle me this one: what part of the body is affected in Charcot-Marie-Tooth disorder? Don't feel bad if you said the teeth - I thought so too!

DISEASE OF THE MONTH

As we all attempt to shove a seemingly insurmountable amount of information between our two ears (and keep it there), different medical students find that certain strategies work best with their learning style: flashcards, question banks, perhaps the textbook-as-a-pillow method.

In my first year of medical school, I can confidently say that the best, and perhaps only way, for me to forever commit a disease process to memory is to convince myself, down to my very core, that I have it.

Luckily, my list of self-diagnoses has taken me on a journey through most of the body's systems. It is rare for me to go a whole unit without coming across a PowerPoint slide that sounds like it was made with me in mind.

From ovarian cancer to colorectal cancer to squamous cell carcinoma of the ear. From an occult inguinal hernia to Lyme disease. Not only have my trials and tribulations motivated me to take deep dives into the literature, through a myriad of medical appointments I have been able to explore specialties I never would have considered otherwise!

Was it worth the late nights spent on Reddit forums where posters analyze each other's pictures of stool? Only time will tell.

SO CLOSE, YET SO FAR

"Yeah so I've been feeling pretty tired recently," our patient recounted.

I leaned back into the counter - my attending had taken the only other chair beside the patient - and sighed as every question I had asked and presented was repeated.

"Uh huh..." My attending mumbled, typing furiously on his computer. It was 4pm on a Friday in Family medicine clinic, and leaving notes for the weekend was not the goal.

"I'm not really sure what's causing it, or when it started really."

I nodded along, eyes glazing, smiling encouragingly from the back of the room.

"Hey you know I think I could have necrophilia?!"

My mind sprang to attention. The clicking of the keyboard came to a stunned halt. My attending spun around in his chair, "I'm sorry, what was that?"

"Necro...wait, wait hang on what does that mean? I think I meant narcolepsy guys?"

"I really hope so, ma'am."

THE RESIDENT SLAYER

Coming into medical school, my parents always told me, "You're not allowed to date until you're a doctor." I figured, I couldn't wait that long – so if I wasn't going to be a doctor soon, maybe I'll just date one!

Let's face it, dating in med school is no piece of cake. The only people you meet are either at school or at the grocery store. But once you enter the hospital for clinical rotations, you meet so many new people. Nurses, PA students, and most importantly, residents.

I thought I had found love in Internal Medicine, but it turns out she doesn't wear her wedding ring to work. On Pediatrics I thought I found the one, only to find out that I'm just too young for her. General Surgery, though, was where I really left my heart. She was brilliant, dedicated, emphatic, and hilarious. For a week I performed the usual detective work to find out that she was in fact single – call me Sherlock Holmes. But before I could ask her on a date, she was switched to another service.

Enough was enough. I really needed to broaden my horizons, and I wasn't a fan of the new nickname my friends were giving me – "The Resident Slayer." A ton of my friends struck gold on dating apps, so I thought I would try my luck. I downloaded everything from Tinder to Bumble, answered a few irrelevant questions, and was ready to put myself out there.

First match: my General Surgery resident. Uh oh. I needed a quick consult to my roommate.

We stared at my phone, trying to come up with an ice-breaker equally filled with wit and acknowledgement of the awkwardness of the situation. Do I go with humor?

Do I make a pun? Do I present a patient? The possibilities were endless.

I sent a message but never received a response. But I didn't feel sad, I just thought one thing:

I sure hope that's not going on my eval.

DIARY OF A MED STUDENT

———

PART THREE

TALES

OF

JOY

———

Life is not measured by the number of breaths we take, but the moments that take our breath away.

— Maya Angelou

Happiness makes up in height for what it lacks in length.

— Robert Frost

If you want to be happy, be.

— Leo Tolstoy

LOVING HER DEARLY

When the love of my life started medical school, I knew she would need all of my support to get through it. I knew this because she told me.

"Sam," she said. "I will need all of your support to get through this."

I smiled, kissed her face, and she stroked my hair the way she always does. "I'm serious," she said. "This will take a lot out of me, and I don't know if I'll be the same person coming out." She turned my head until her eyes leveled with mine. "Don't lose me, okay?"

I nodded in agreement. But I didn't know how much that would entail.

"I love you," she'd say in the morning. "I'll see you when I get back."

I never know when she'll be back.

There are long days, days when I find myself waiting for her to return, running in circles, almost driving myself crazy with worry. Is this worth it? Who am I? Who is that strange man coming to the doorbell? What if she leaves me for someone else? She never does, though.

There are days when I know she'd be too tired to cook. I wish I could cook; I wish I could cook so badly to make her happy. But I don't know how. One time I gathered my favorite things for her to eat. She picked through it, smiled politely, and made both of us dinner.

I wish I could cook, so that I can love her more.

There are days when she cries. These are the days when she needs me the most, to listen, to just be there. Days before exams.

Days after exams.

We don't lie in bed and cuddle anymore like we used to. There is no more time for that.

We have fights.

"Let's go out," I'd say. "We should really go out, blow off some steam. Come on, we'll have a ball."

"I can't. I have Renal."

"Rough."

I knew that she would be suffering, but to this extent, I did not know. Her mind wanders; am I losing her?

Never. Her heart is tethered on a leash to mine.

During these times, I can only wag my tail, await her return, and give her all of my love.

It's the best a dog can do.

A LITTLE SHORT

Contrary to popular belief, medical school is filled with joy, and for many of us, that joy originates from getting our white coats.

Yet, the joy from receiving the white coat does not always permeate the entire ceremony. For me, we had already rehearsed the ceremony once. We had just been standing in a single-file line in blistering heat. And now we had the pleasure of listening to multiple speeches that all seemed to last a little too long.

But once the first student received their coat, my butterflies started flying. As the line in front of me shortened, I thought of all the times that took me to this moment. Studying for the MCAT for what felt like 30 hours a day. Taking my first blood pressure on the wrong arm. Revising my personal statement more times than should be legal.

When it was my turn, all those feelings went away. I put my arm through one sleeve, then the other, and finally puffed out my chest in a way that would make any bodybuilder proud. Though there were hundreds of people in the auditorium that night, during that moment, it felt like a spotlight came down on my family. For a split second, it was just them and me in the room.

During the after-ceremony reception, I was overcome with the expected congratulatory comments and hugs from my parents. But as is tradition, my brother broke the ice: "Nice job, but why is your white coat so short?"

Still smiling, I looked down at my shiny new armor. He was right, it did look a little short.

Perhaps it was because the white coat was a bit small.

Or perhaps, it was because I was standing a little bit taller.

BUTTERFLIES

Chief complaint: "butterflies" in stomach

General: excitable
Cardiovascular: elevated heart rate
Pulmonary: elevated respiratory rate
Eyes: widened bilaterally

History: It was only 60 seconds prior that I had an unread email in my inbox titled "Admissions Decision," and clicking that would induce the above symptoms.

Assessment: Incredibly grateful to be accepted into medical school. A bit nervous as I know the road ahead will not be easy, but excited for what the future holds.

Plan: To be competent in my work, curious in my investigation, creative in my approach, and compassionate to my patients as I strive to become the best doctor I can be.

—

Follow-up: So much has happened in one year. I've learned about the heart in lecture, dissected it in anatomy, and listened to it in clinic. I memorized over 1,000 flashcards facts one day, and helped over 10 patients another day. Some days I'm exhausted from all the work. Other days I am indomitable. Each day of medical school for has been entirely unique—the only constant after one year is that my "butterflies" of excitement persist, each and every day.

MY GRANDMA IS IN YOUR ANATOMY LAB

The night before my first anatomy lab was fraught with anxiety, even more so than it is for most medical students.

Three months earlier, my beloved grandma had died, after a long and happy life filled with love and connection. The next day, my dad called to say that he and my uncles thought it might be a good idea to donate her body to science; I agreed. Then, he said, "And guess where she's going?"

Sure enough, Grandma's body was going to a particular medical school – the school I had committed to attending just weeks before.

Though the anatomy department had assured us that I would never come in contact with her body, as our first lab approached, both typical and unique fears surfaced for me. Would I pass out at the first incision? Would my group get along? What if they gave me Grandma's body by mistake? What if dissecting another human body made me think too much about what would happen to hers?

As it turned out, my cadaver was a man, my group became friends, I stayed vertical the whole time, and as the weeks went on, anatomy lab became a special and joyful experience for me – in part thanks to Grandma.

I was acutely aware that the body I was dissecting had once been someone else's grandpa, uncle, friend, or cousin, which inspired a very real sense of respect. Still, I was happy to find that all of my classmates treated their cadavers with the same sense of dignity and awe – I am lucky to be surrounded by these people.

As dissection became more routine, and the mood in lab lightened, my group often started to chat, laugh, and poke fun at our professors as the afternoon passed, and I had the strong sense that this was okay. Grandma had a great sense of humor, and she loved being the center of attention; I know she would have been very comfortable in this happy environment, even postmortem.

Grandma knew I was starting medical school, and she knew which school I was going to, but toward the end of her life she had become a little forgetful, and I wasn't sure if she remembered those facts when she died. I began to find a deep and totally unscientific sense of contentment in a feeling that because her body was right next door, she really knew where I was.

Best of all, as my dad said, he liked the idea of being able to tell people that he was sending his daughter AND his mother to medical school.

The joy Grandma brought to my life is stronger than ever.

"IF YOU HIT THE SKULL, YOU'VE GONE TOO FAR!"

"My preceptor lets me do everything," I liked to brag. Now I stood there, getting ready to do a punch biopsy for the first time, feeling both the circular blade in my hand and a deep feeling of uncertainty.

The patient and my preceptor were both completely unfazed. For my preceptor, it was a "probably nothing," ho-hum kind of lesion which we would take out and send to pathology anyway. For the patient, who was a jovial veteran, well, he had seen worse things than me.

But for myself, it felt like the first time I got behind the wheel of a car. It was night in a large parking lot, and my dad had taken me there to "try driving" before I started driver's ed the next day. I remember pressing the gas timidly and feeling a lurch as the car jerked suddenly forward, too fast. "We're not driving lawn mowers anymore, Toto."

"How deep should I go?" I had asked my preceptor outside of the room, buying time.

"Well," my preceptor chuckled in his booming voice, waving his large, expressive hands, "If you hit skull, you've gone too far!"

This sounds like an unhelpful answer, but if I'm being honest, I'm no good at estimating distances anyway. Had he said something specific like "2 centimeters," then I would have had cause to panic. As it stood, I was left with the impression that it didn't matter much. Maybe.

Well, I wasn't going to get any more ready. I pressed the blade against the patient's skull, twisting several times, to get to the deeply technical depth of "arbitrary," before pulling out. Then I used scissors to snip out what I had cut loose, dropped it in the pathology cup, and sewed the patient's small wound shut.

The patient wasn't bleeding out and was still making jokes. My preceptor was still smiling. I guess that means it worked.

Maybe I'll get lucky next time too.

BAND-AIDS AND SUTURES

I taught myself how to suture a few years ago with a pilfered kit and some Prolene I bought from a veterinary supplier on the internet. I sewed up an orange peel and posted a picture of it with a witty caption. I was pretty proud of myself.

The first time I sutured on a real live human was different. It was the middle of the night and the patient was a crying kindergartener who didn't speak a lot of English and wasn't interested enough to try to understand my attempt at comforting Spanish. She had smashed her tiny pinky finger in a door, which left her with a fractured bone and a big laceration underneath her magenta-painted fingernail. With my attending's guidance, it was my job to remove the nail, sew up the laceration, and then replace the nail and glue it down.

Oranges are a lot bigger than the pinky nail beds of 5-year-olds. I was pleasantly surprised to see my needle pierce the necessary tissue and to see the jagged edges of the cut come together so well as I tied my first knot. The holes I had made bled, making me worry that maybe I had done something wrong, but I mopped up the blood and finished the job. Once the nail was back in place and we had talked to the family about wound care, we left the nurse to bandage the finger so we could put in discharge papers.

As we were getting ready to send our patient home, the nurse came to ask if we could come back, saying the patient was in a lot of pain. Immediately, I felt guilty and wracked my brain for what had gone wrong. Did I push the nail back in too far? Did I drive the needle too deep and disrupt the fracture? I was terrified that my inexperience and lack of expertise had caused this little girl and her family unnecessary pain and maybe even mistrust in our hospital. I stood behind my attending while she examined that little pinky and my work, positive that I was about to watch the physician tell the family that the procedure would need to be redone.

But then, the doctor asked the patient if she wanted a popsicle. The inconsolable sobbing paused. And then we offered her a Band-Aid. In that moment, a weight lifted and I jumped in to ask what color she wanted. I unwrapped her choice and carefully covered up my work. The crying stopped altogether. Things suddenly felt better. I hadn't messed up.

We talk a lot about Band-Aids being a symbol for an inadequate and temporary solution to a problem. But in the right situation, as it turns out, a hot pink Band-Aid really can make all the difference.

SEE ONE, DO ONE, TEACH ONE

On my emergency medicine rotation, it was clear that the "see one, do one, teach one" adage really applied. We had a patient who came in for dizziness and nausea due to BPPV.

"Have you ever done an Epley maneuver on someone?" said my senior resident.

Without a beat, I replied, "Nope, but I can learn!"

"Great! Here's a YouTube video you can watch. After, go ahead and try it on the patient and then let me know how it goes. It probably won't work, but you can try."

I knew what the Epley maneuver was and the concept of it, but I did not remember all the exact steps to do it. I excitedly watched the video and committed the coordinated dance moves to memory. It sort of is reminiscent of ballroom dancing if you think about it...the patient moves one way, and then I guide the patient's head with my hands another way...

After rehearsing the moves I had just watched on an imaginary patient in front of me in the workroom, I sprung up and went straight to the patient's room before I forgot all the steps and directions. I explained to her what I would be doing as confidently as I could as if I had done this multiple times and it was not my very first time doing the maneuver on a real patient. She, and her husband with her in the room, looked at me half-skeptically but agreed to try it to alleviate her symptoms.

The nausea and dizziness were still there after the first try and only partially went away after the second try. I was beginning to lose hope and share the same doubtfulness to the maneuver as the resident did.

However, after the next try, I asked again if she still had nausea afterwards. She, to my surprise, cracked her first smile of the encounter, and shook her head. Had it really worked?! Was my success rate with the Epley maneuver really at a whopping 100%?! 1 for 1! I taught her and her husband the Epley maneuver in case they wanted to try it on their own at home too. See one, do one, teach one.

I reported back to the resident, who had the same doubts as I did, but that was about all we could do at the time regardless. I kept thinking to myself, did the patient really gain relief with the maneuver? Or did she just tell me that to make me stop asking her to lay down quickly, turn her head, hold it there, sit up, etc... Either way, for all intents and purposes, it worked and she was discharged.

NOT BAD FOR A FIRST YEAR

Nerves wracked my body. Deep breath in. Deep breath out. Ok, you can handle a night shift in the ED. One foot in front of another and the automatic doors separated from each other.

The emergency department was daunting. The waiting room was filled. Despair and frustration was palpable. I hoped that my short white coat was enough of a difference from the residents and attendings. I couldn't possibly know enough to help them yet. With my head down and quick strides, I escaped the waiting room unscathed.

I was amazed. The rapid-fire questions from the physicians quickly narrowed down the diagnosis and a plan of action was finalized minutes later. As a first year, my rudimentary interviewing skills with standardized patients felt like a completely different practice.

I was flustered. When a resident wanted me to hear a patient's murmur, my stethoscope was hesitantly placed on the woman's skin. Blood rushed to my face when he moved it to the correct location.

I was exasperated. All the studying for my cardiology exam seemed like a distant memory when an attending handed me an EKG. My blank stare answered her question if I could assess the patient's condition. I was way out of my league.

The physician I was shadowing encouraged me to ask any questions I had. I had none. I didn't even know what I didn't know. It was going to be a long eight hours.

Slowly, my observations and anticipation allowed me to assimilate into the demanding dynamic of the emergency department. I identified atrial fibrillation on an EKG. I assisted a resident draining an abscess. I joined the fourth-year medical students performing E-FAST scans. By the end of the night, I completed the ultrasound scans by myself, with the fourth years cheering me on. One of them whooped: "Hey! Not bad for a first year!" I couldn't help the Cheshire cat grin that spread across my face.

Morning was coming and I should have been yearning for caffeine. But I was humming; humming with a purpose. The long nights studying, the many applications, and the grueling pressure gained more perspective than they ever had. I completed all these tasks with the broader picture in mind, but finally I was able to taste a little bit of this purpose. I was invigorated.

The rest of the eight hours flew by and as I was leaving, the intense waiting room did not seem so scary anymore. Head held high, my feet carried me into the crisp morning air, excited to study following a nice nap. Not bad for a first year, indeed.

TAKING THE CALL

The call I had been waiting for came in around 11:00 AM, just as I got home from the hospital. This was my third-year surgery rotation, and after many days of early mornings reviewing charts and holding various instruments in the OR for what felt like hours, I knew opportunities like this were rare.

"Hey, do you still want to help with the BKA (below-knee amputation) going this morning?" the surgical intern asked.

"YES," I said without hesitation.

"Well, it's rolling back in 15 minutes so hurry."

On AM rounds earlier, the residents had mentioned a patient may need a BKA to control possible spread of infection from dry gangrene to his right foot. I had just come off mandatory night call, so part of me was looking forward to my day off. That was until the chief told me I could help if the surgery went.

"No [insert expletive] way" I thought as the resident described how the surgery would be a guillotine amputation using a metal wire. A word of advice he gave was "Once you start, don't stop until the limb is off."

Those words rang in my head as I rushed back to the hospital and found the right OR. The chief resident looked surprised to see me. AM rounds had finished at 8am, and I had already stuck around for three additional hours before deciding to head home. I was here now though, and the attending handed me the wire as the patient was put under anesthesia. He walked me through how I would need to use a "see-saw" type motion and pimped me lightly on what the three major vessels were that I would encounter bleeding from. Finally, he echoed what the chief had told me earlier and said, "Once you start, don't stop until the limb is off."

I braced myself under the incision line and went for it using that "see-saw" motion. After what felt like a blink, I had just performed my first BKA as a medical student! Bleeding started happening immediately, and in the moment, I was even given the Bovie to cauterize those three vessels! The case finished shortly after, and the resident and attending told me "good job."

I returned home to enjoy my day, glad I had taken that phone call. As a medical student, these opportunities come along rarely. So, it does not matter if you are post-call or tired from waiting around three hours after rounds or literally sitting on the toilet thinking "They probably won't call." Take the opportunity. You may end up with a pretty good story to tell.

MY FIRST CIRCUMCISION

Newborn nursery rotation as a 3rd year medical student was a beautiful week of celebrating new life. It was spoiled only by the tribulation of my first circumcision, where everything that could go wrong, did.

Chaos on the floor pulled my attending away. At 5pm, my blood sugar wavered somewhere between hangry and hypoglycemic. The baby whose prepuce I was tasked with removing had the most circuitous raphe any of us had ever seen, obscuring all the usual landmarks. The child began screaming before ever being touched despite our best efforts to soothe him. And, my senior resident, fluent in three languages, forgot how to speak English, instead giving me the instructions "And then... You just... You know..."

I felt overwhelmed, inadequate, and doomed to failure. How was I so unskilled that I couldn't manage this baby's catawampus penis, calm his screams, and interpret my resident's nebulous directions? Internally dying from stress and vicious self-beratement, I was certain that this was the time where I proved I wasn't good enough to be a doctor.

The ordeal lasted for 30 minutes. Everyone survived. My senior complimented my steady hands and grace under pressure. Despite an outcome that most would call a success, I left the hospital and cried for an hour. Doctors are supposed to be perfect, right? Calm, capable; wielding medical knowledge that rivals Google; immune to hunger, fatigue, or mistakes. Against that superhuman requirement, any inadequacy proves my unworthiness. Right?

For years, I didn't know how to be content with imperfection, but I've come to realize that's not fair. It's not fair to myself to expect a flawlessness impossible for the human race. It's not fair to those behind me to endorse such an unhealthy standard. It's not fair to my patients to offer only 100% of me or nothing, when 99% is still phenomenal and improves lives.

If doctors have to be perfect, then there will be no doctors. We will never be perfect. We will make mistakes, continually learn, and need to apologize, but we will still be good doctors, not in spite of our humanity, but because of it. I hope we all have a similar persona-shattering experience that reminds us of our humanity, reignites our pursuit of greatness and compassion, and pushes back the perfectionism that threatens to hold us down. Or maybe many of them, because we're stubborn and don't learn these kinds of lessons easily.

KITCHEN DECISION

I began interviewing our newly admitted patient, a 60 or so year-old rugged gentleman hospitalized for something less important than his next remark.

"I used to be a major smoker, like a 2-pack-a-day kind of guy. But I went from that to none last year," to which I congratulated him excitedly. I was quite impressed as I have tried motivating many patients to quit before, with varied success; I was truly curious to his secret. He went on to say how he tried to quit for years without any luck. His family was hard on him for his smoking habits, including his wife who cried several times because of his worsening respiratory symptoms. "Even with all that, I still had no luck with trying to quit," he continued.

Until one day. He came home to see his wife in the kitchen... "Uh oh!" I thought, "That's never a good sign." His wife had never smoked before, yet here she was lighting one up in the kitchen. And not only that, there were 5 or so finished cigarettes in the ashtray from earlier in the day. His wife said, "I can't change you, so I'm going with your flow and will try to keep up until whatever happens."

He then looks up at me and says, "And that's the last day I ever smoked."

This struck me as one of the realest love stories that I've ever heard. All the visits doctors spent with him reciting the health risks of smoking proved fruitless; the greatest medicine of all for him was love. It's incredible the changes patients make in their lives when we dig beneath the surface to find a personal way to self-motivate them. For him, the old adage rang true: happy wife, happy life.

GET UP AND GO

I had a patient complete a Get Up and Go Test today, a screening test for patients at risk for falling. It is quite a simple test with a self-explanatory name. My patient was amicable, kind, and loved to give me advice she would have given her younger self if she could.

I explained the process of the test and she completed it with flying colors. We settled back down into our seats and I knew I was about to get an earful by the look on her face.

"That was quite a silly test," she chuckled, "I'm glad I passed by just living." I smiled as she continued to reflect. "I see you knuckle heads are worried about me bumbling around at home but that is just a part of life. I'm fine. We fall, sure, but then we get right back up do exactly what your little test says, and go." I was taken aback. What a grand metaphor!

True, this screening test's clinical application is a bit more serious, but its name provides great life advice nonetheless. In life, we really are just stumbling about. It is unpredictable and we face challenges everyday no matter how prepared we are. We fall and we get back up. We try and we fail. We make mistakes and we learn from them. Importantly, even if only because there is no other option, we keep going.

Medical school is no easy path. There are plenty of times where I felt I hit rock bottom or that I may never recover. There were times when I felt like an imposter, like I would never be good enough. There were times when I fell and struggled to pick myself back up.

But then I did. In the end, I always got back up. I had a goal and I wouldn't let anything hold me down. I had to get back up and I had to keep going.

Life may be a bit more uncertain and falls less easily predicted than with a medical screening tool. But I think our strength lies in the ability to continue to get up and go despite the struggles. Especially our patients, the ones who push up from a chair with ever muscle in their body. The ones who walk with their head high as they slowly shuffle down the hallway. They are the ones who inspire us to keep going.

Because in life we may stumble and we may have falls, but after a moment of recovery we still get up and go. I will continue to go. Despite challenges and seemingly insurmountable falls, I will go. And I implore you, please go with me.

THE FRUITS OF HER LABOR

I arrived at morning report on Labor & Delivery as the charge nurse reviewed the list. "Med student, you're taking the lead in room 9. The mother is very anxious— her last delivery was a crash section." I wondered "is she talking to me?" I was confused, scared, and excited. As the lone student on the service, I followed every patient on the floor; however, I had never been in charge of a patient. It was time to show everyone that I could do more than just get in the way.

I reviewed the patient's chart and reviewed c-sections, making sure that I could answer every question my patient could ask me. I did my Wonder Woman pose and went to room 9. I knocked on the door and introduced myself, eager to spew all my obstetrical knowledge.

Before I could ask my patient if she had any questions, she asked if I could just sit with her and talk. Confused, I sat down. We talked about her life, hobbies, and aspirations. It seems so simple now, but this mother had a life outside of the few hours I got to interact with her. She was not just a patient, but she was a person.

When it was time to roll back to the OR, she grabbed my hand and asked if I was coming with her. Once again, I found myself wondering "is she talking to me?" I had spent the past several years diligently memorizing facts and learning pathways to become the best doctor I could be; however, it was in this moment that I learned what it truly meant to be a physician. It wasn't just about grades and board scores, but it was the ability to make an impact on someone's life and guide them through their vulnerable medical experiences. Although my patient told me that I helped her through her delivery, what she doesn't know is how much she helped me.

THE HEIGHT OF MY TRAINING

Of all the joyous moments in medical school, the days I spent on sports medicine were my favorite. I was a rookie medic – not the kind that a pro soccer player wants to see when he tears an ACL. Yet here I was, hanging out in the big leagues as I rotated through major sporting events. This memorable morning, I packed my first aid kit, threw in an extra tube of Neosporin for good measure, and went on my way to help with the physicals for a famous professional soccer team.

As any med student would, I made sure to get there before my attendings' alarm clocks had even rung. Soon enough, the big-shot doctors walked in. We gathered in a circle, and began the ritual of introducing ourselves to the team one by one. Luckily, I was last.

"Hi, my name is so and so. Head physician of the NFL team so and so." A round of applause and cheers. Huh, guess he's out of my league.

"Hi, I'm so and so, head of orthopaedic surgery for the NBA team so and so." A louder round of applause, more cheers. It was starting to look like passing out coffee might be all I can offer here.

Needless to say, I didn't get a standing ovation when I introduced myself as 4th year medical student. Nevertheless, they gave me the most important job of all: checking every player's height. I could pinch myself; I was here alongside my heroes serving famous athletes – nothing could be better! I began banging out these height checks like clockwork. And like any good medical student would, I pulled out my Anki cards and flipped through them between patients.

Now here's the thing. I love soccer and played all my life, and I really admire the players for how hard they work. Yet, I couldn't name a single player on this entire team, and I was too busy swiping through my sports med Ankis the night before to look up any of the players' names before the event! My friends had all told me, "You GOTTA get an autograph from player DM!" Perfect, I know his last name but I got no clue what he looks like. So, I waited and waited. Each player would come up and introduce himself...Nope that's not his name.

Then finally... a player came up to me and introduced himself by FIRST NAME ONLY. I'm thinking maybe that's him, but if it's not then I'll waste my one napkin on the wrong autograph! I wasn't 100% sure if he was the player so I casually checked his height and directed him to the next station.

After the event, I put in a STAT consult in to Dr. Google. Assessment: Yes, he was in fact the player. Plan: never again miss a chance like that over a couple of Anki cards. Even though I did not get the autograph, it was one of my favorite days of med school! And who knows, maybe I'll get to come back one day. Only next time I won't be introducing myself as MS4.

THE LITTLE I COULD OFFER

It was early Saturday morning as we neared the end of our rounding list when we entered Ms. K's room. She was 24 hours into her recovery, and was already awake and reading, her foot bobbing off the side of the bed metronomically. She thanked the team profusely for the prior day's operation. But as we told her the brief plan of continuing pain control, ambulating, and advancing her diet, her facial expression shifted and her foot stilled.

"Hey... umm is there any way of knowing how much small bowel they had to take yesterday? Or how much is left?" Ms. K inquired with hesitation, half stumbling on her words.

"I'm sorry, but I wasn't the surgeon that did your operation" the attending hastily replied, halfway out the doorway. I looked back as we filed out of the room; Ms. K now sat on her bed, her head down, legs frozen.

I circled back to visit Ms. K after the last patient was rounded on. She explained to me that she used to work for the Department of Public Health and was very familiar with PubMed and other medical literature that she had access to through her career. Up until her battle with ovarian cancer, Ms. K had found her health literacy a helpful tool – she struggled with anxiety and her main coping mechanism was to learn more about whatever was causing her stress. However, now she was in a position where the EHR system and surgeons possessed the information that would help her. Her treatment was inaccessible.

"I'm not worried about getting bad news, I just want to know where I stand so I can start planning and envisioning my future... I feel unprepared. I'm a nervous wreck. I can't accept a new normal without knowing what that new normal will entail. Not knowing is driving me up the wall" Ms. K said, her voice crescendoing with emotion.

We sat together for a moment in silence, and then I had an idea. My fingers pecked at the keyboard as I logged into the EHR system.

"I'm only a medical student, but how about I pull up the note from the operation and we can see what your surgeon said?"

Ms. K's face lit up with excitement. The little I could offer, was the little that she needed. I opened the note and she began to read, her foot bobbing once again.

WAKE UP THE WARRIORS!

"We gave Molly the Neupogen shot, but it took 2 residents, 2 nurses, and her mom holding her down while she fought against us." I listened with a blend of amusement and horror as the night team relayed the grand efforts it took to give one shot to a fierce little girl who absolutely hated needles.

Molly was an 8-year old with a complex medical history who was in the hospital because her white blood cells were dangerously low, so much so that even the most harmless bacteria could cause a life-threatening illness. The Neupogen shots would stimulate her bone marrow to produce more white blood cells so that she'd be safe to go home.

During rounds that morning, I learned that Molly's white blood cells had an encouraging rise in response to the shot, and she would be sent home that day. But Molly would need another shot to be administered by her parents at home. How will her mother react when I tell her she'll need 4 people and a nurse's skill level to deliver the shot?

Molly and her mom's faces went through a full spectrum of emotions as I let them know first the good news, then the bad. "NO SHOTS!" Molly screamed repeatedly, tears rolling down her cheeks. As a medical student, I had one secret weapon that no one else on my team had – time. I pulled up a chair and tried to level with her.

"Has anyone explained to you why you need these shots?" Molly shook her head no. "Everyone is just trying to hurt me!"

"Of course not!" I exclaimed. I proceeded to tell her a story about white blood cell warriors that fight off the bad guy germs that get kids sick. I told her how her warriors were asleep, and these shots would help wake them up so she wouldn't get sick again.

Molly looked at me skeptically. "Are you sure the shot will wake up my warriors?" she asked.

"Well, it sure woke them up last night, didn't it?" I retorted. Molly pondered this for a second, eyes widening as she put her little hand on her chin, and said "That's true. I want my warriors to wake up!" Molly's mom thanked me as I left the room for helping reduce her daughter's resistance to shots, even if just a little bit.

I had a bounce in my step as I walked out of Molly's room that day. It felt amazing to be able to make this little girl feel included in her own care. Though saying goodbye was hard, I knew Molly would be safe at home. She had an army of warriors behind her.

CLOUDY BREAKS

"My sister passed last week," said Ms. A, as tears began to fall. "I'm sorry," said the doctor, glancing at her with tender eyes. I stood there, ingesting the aura of authentic connection between healer and sufferer. A first-year medical student, I had no medical acumen – but I knew empathy, and here it was.

Yet the glance – the empathy – was just a glance. "So, let's talk about your blood pressure." Ms. A didn't bring up her sister one more time after that. Through a continual stream of tears, she answered the doctor's series of questions about her physical health, punctuated by another "I'm sorry" from the doctor when Ms. A's grief momentarily interrupted her train of thought. The encounter drew to a close, and the doctor left the room.

Ms. A grabbed her purse and prepared to rise from her chair when I sat down beside her and asked, "Can we talk more about your sister?" "We were so close," she said.

"Tell me more."

For the first time this visit, I could see Ms. A relax a bit in her chair. She had a strong familial support system, she said, but it was still an emotional toil for everyone. I asked her if she had received or sought grief counseling. "No," she said.

"Would you like us to connect you with someone to talk to?"

"Yes, I think I would like that," she said.

At the front desk, the receptionist referred her to a social worker. I waited until the last minute to make sure this actually happened.

I don't know if Ms. A ever connected with the social worker. I wish I had followed up with her. Instead, I got lost in my studies – about the physical body and its diseases – and forgot all about it. When I think back to that day, I am not sad, upset, or regretful. Instead, I am joyful.

I am joyful that Ms. A did not leave the office without having a chance to talk with someone, even briefly, about what was clearly the most important thing on her mind.

I am joyful that she was given the chance to follow-up with someone who could help her process and heal from her grief.

I am joyful that even as a medical student who knew virtually nothing about how to treat her ongoing health problems, I could still impact her healthcare.

There are many dark days in medical school, but the cloudy breaks often seem to arrive at just the right time. And I rejoice in them.

I DON'T KNOW

"I don't know," my preceptor, Dr. G, said to her patient presenting with nonspecific abdominal pain. A first-year medical student, I stood in the corner and condensed into as little space as possible as my widened eyes darted between physician and patient. Among a schedule chock-full of lectures, small group sessions, and extracurricular meetings, this was my biweekly half-day to observe my mentor, an internal medicine physician in my city's community. We were reaching the end of one of several, 15-minute-long patient visits for the day; I'd already observed numerous greetings, thorough histories, and meticulous physical exams, each concluding precisely on time with an assessment and plan. Two whole minutes past this visit's allotted duration, however, Dr. G uttered the one phrase I'd thought was banned from a physician's glossary.

Upon entering medical school, I was stunned, as many are, at the volume of information presented to me. As a recovering perfectionist, I take issue with the inevitability of letting details slip through the cracks. What's an appropriate level of slippage? Can I do this? Do I belong here? Imposter syndrome consumed me. As I reflect now, with one academic year under my belt, I feel unsatisfied with the amount of time I spent degrading my efforts. My post-exam ritual seemed to involve berating myself for a lack of perfection rather than taking pride in my achievement. During these times, my emotions forced logical thinking onto the back burner.

Just hearing my preceptor's "I don't know" represented a significant realization for me during my medical career, and I'm grateful that this turning point happened as early as it did. In that moment, Dr. G humanized medicine. Physicians are ultra-respected in the community, and I fiercely defend their reputations. At times, however, I feel like a novice outsider constantly groveling at the feet of idols whose expertise I've convinced myself I will never attain.

"I don't know" means that I am human. I am trying my best. I believe that my colleagues are, too. I deserve to be here. I'm not expected to do, be, and know everything. I have friendships, hobbies, strengths, and weaknesses. I will act in my role until this role feels natural; I trust that it soon will. In my future practice, I will be humble enough to use "I don't know." I will be vulnerable. I will feel my patients' emotions. I will never quit learning. I will repeat these statements. These are the principles by which I will live.

SMALL MOMENTS

On the second to last day of my neurology rotation, amidst the scrambling of last minute practice questions for the looming next-day shelf, I was asked to see a new patient. I walked into the exam room knowing only that he had had some trouble maintaining his balance for a few weeks. My hearty greeting was met with a pungent cloud of cigarette butts, urine, and body odor.

In front of me sat a smiling, disheveled man. His hair long and tangled. His hands rough. His nails dirty. For the next 15 minutes, we talked, I prodded, and he struggled to take his sneakers off to show me his feet. He was a pleasure to interview, our senses of humor were similar, and we took turns asking questions and listening intently to what the other person had to share. When I guessed the symptoms he'd forgotten to mention, his face lit up and he clapped – yes, he also had that! How did I know?

I left to report to my attending, returning shortly thereafter. In the middle of the doctor's explanation, the man interrupted. He pointed at me with his dusky finger, and said, "your assistant here is really good, doc, she got everything right. You should keep her around."

I straightened my back a few degrees, puffed out my chest an inch, and couldn't contain the red rushing to my cheeks.

"Tomorrow's her last day so I can't do that, but I wish I could too."

I glanced at my usually stoic attending – surprised – and smiled as the stress melted away for a few moments. I was proud.

THE SILENT WAR

"Oh that was easy" "not too bad" everyone says
But as I remember my struggle with the test
The question lingers "Do I fit in with the rest?"
I worked hard to get where I am
But is this supposed to be part of the plan?
"You'll get the hang of it" they say
How can that be if I don't even know the way?
As my classmates get together in clusters
Enjoying lectures, having fun
I ask myself, maybe I am an imposter?
Maybe I am the only one?
I wake up and realize,
These thoughts have come up again before my eyes.
I stare into the ceiling like a deer in headlights,
Trying to remove these feelings like it's a life or death
fight.
I wipe away the salty taste from my tears,
As my amygdala amplifies my fears.
My tachycardia relaxes,
As I remove these mental axes.
While getting ready I catch a glimpse in the mirror
White coat, stethoscope and pen light too.
Realization kicks in and I ask, "can this really be true?"
"YES!" my heart exclaims
Being the wielder of my pains.
"You're meant for this and so much more"
I gain courage and I lift up my gaze from the floor.
As my heart overpowers my brain,
I look at the path that's been laid.
I knock at the door, a voice says "come in"
I greet the patient, "Welcome to my office, let's begin."
The struggle is real, the end is worth fighting for,
never relinquish, never call defeat
in this never-ending silent war.

DIARY OF A MED STUDENT

PART FOUR

TALES

OF

INSPIRATION

Once you have tasted flight, you will
forever walk the earth with your eyes
turned skyward, for there you have been,
and there you will always long to return.
                                    – Leonardo da Vinci

It does not matter how slowly you go
as long as you do not stop.
                                    – Confucius

Isn't it nice to think that tomorrow
is a new day with no mistakes in it yet?
                                    – L.M. Montgomery

NO MATTER WHAT

The first thing I did on Wednesday November 9, 2016 was quickly check my phone for the election results. I had gone to bed late even though I had to wake up early for my clinical day at the Charlestown Clinic. Nevertheless, I fell asleep without knowing who the next President of the United States would be. Upon seeing the result, a feeling of dread fell over me. Nevertheless, I told myself to make sure to keep it together during the day at clinic, and that I would have time later to process.

The clinical day began smoothly, with multiple positive educational experiences.

Then one particular patient, an elderly man coming into clinic with his adult son, suddenly changed the course of the morning. The older man wore a Trump shirt. The front read "Make America Great Again" and the back displayed a misogynistic image and slur.

Upon entering the examination room, I immediately felt many different emotions. As an under-represented minority student in medicine, I felt unwelcomed and unsafe. I felt anger at what I considered to be a smug and offensive display on the patient's shirt.

Multiple power dynamics were simultaneously at play in the room. Some hierarchies in their favor – two bulky, tattooed white men in a room with a woman of color attending physician and two Latinx medical students. However, I realized quickly that the patient was powerless in a different way.

During the early encounter, I tried to find compassion in my heart. "We treat patients, no matter what," I told myself. "We heal, no matter what." Then, it became clear from the conversation in the room that this older man was fighting cancer. His cancer had metastasized, and this was causing a great deal of suffering. He eventually broke down in tears in front of us all as he became overwhelmed with his situation.

My feelings of frustration and anger soon gave way to feelings of shame. I was so quick to judge the man before me. Initially, I failed to see him with the empathy and compassion of a caring clinician. I reflected on how my biases, explicit or implicit, could seriously impact the care I provide in future years.

As soon as this visit ended and the patient left, my preceptor broke down in tears. Based on the few words she said to my classmate and me, I realized she may have been going through an internal conversation similar to mine. Less than a minute after she began crying, abruptly, she composed herself and entered the next patient chart to prepare for the next visit.

HAND IN HAND

"Would you like a hand massage?" I asked the frail, elderly woman. She was lying in a hospital bed with one arm hooked up to a dialysis machine. As she turned her attention from the small TV screen, she said, "I have never received a massage, but sure." That was not the first time I had received such an answer. Most patients I met in the dialysis unit had never received a massage in their life.

"That's okay. It is a pleasure to be able to give you your first!" I enthusiastically stated as I pulled a stool next to her. I carefully took her hand into my mine, noticing the swelling in her palms and fingers and the heaviness of her hand. Her skin was wrinkled with patches of dry red rashes. She also had a swan neck deformity in her third digit, to which I paid extra attention. With non-allergenic lotion, I gently stroked her palm in a circular fashion using the tips of my two thumbs.

Attempting to turn this recently met stranger into a new friend, I began conversing. "Do you have any family?" I asked. "I have a sister and mother, but no family of my own. Never met Mr. Perfect," she apathetically stated. It was difficult to read this patient as the one-sided conversation continued. "Do you mind me asking why you are on dialysis?" I questioned. "My heart medications damaged my kidneys," she stated with an unmoved voice. I was moved, however. Her situation was just another reminder that while we strive for perfection in medicine, medicine is still imperfect. In hopes to cure one disease, another is sometimes created. "I am sorry to hear to that," I sympathetically said.

Trying to change the topic to something more lighthearted, I asked, "Where would you like to travel to?" I regretted asking the question as soon as she responded. "I have never left the country, but I would like to go to Europe. Traveling is difficult because I cannot walk. I have spina bifida." My heart sunk, and my eyes closed. Feeling terrible for asking all the seemingly wrong questions, I decided to stop questioning. In silence, I continued to massage her palm and fingers with the repeating five strokes I knew, attending to each unique line and crease.

When an hour had passed, I began collecting my items to move on to the next patient. My mind still felt heavy with sadness and guilt. Wishing the patient my best wishes, I stood up to walk away. As I turned by back, I heard her soft voice behind me. "Actually, can you massage my other hand too?" I smiled and said, "It would be my pleasure."

STILL ALICE

Have you ever seen "Still Alice (2014)"?
I met an Alice today.

The doctor and I entered the room and introduced ourselves. Alice had a broad smile on her face; her eyes twinkling on the exam table. As the reflex hammer struck her knees, she swung her arms reflexively and laughed out loud with such child-like exuberance.

The doctor pointed at the gentleman by her side and asked Alice who it was.
Alice replied sweetly, "my husband," - she doesn't know his name.
Then she followed with, "But WHO IS THAT?" pointing at the young boy sitting by her husband.
That was her son.

I thought I could hear my own heart break, against her son's glassy eyes.

Alice was diagnosed with early-onset Alzheimer's when she was 61 years old, earlier than the average age. She used to be a high-functioning individual, a "Power Woman." She now chattered with me as if I were her long-lost friend, telling me that she loves her husband so much - for the tenth time now. She nodded and shook her head along every time a medication was talked about. She asked if I thought the young boy was handsome because her own son is handsome just like him.

"I am so happy!" She exclaims. And she smiles on.

No, I could not envision the electricity that dances through her neuronal tangles, nor could I imagine the thoughts that race through her family's minds. I could barely hold on to my own emotion, thinking what if this were me, or if she were my mom.

What I wish, perhaps naively, is that Alice IS happy. Perhaps this is selfish of me, to want to believe she simply regressed to her carefree childhood; to believe that her son built a fortress around his heart.

But at that moment, I understood one thing, as Maya Angelou wrote, "nothing can dim the light which shines from within." Nothing. She is Alice. She is Still Alice – and she always will be.

THE TIES THAT BIND

When I met Grace, I was a fearful, striving medical student. Grace was the first patient to ask me about my day, and as cliché as it sounds, meeting her changed my life.

Grace was on dialysis and had cancer, and eventually during her stay we held a family meeting. Despite the short notice, her relatives crowded the family room. And there she was, in a scene so perfect it seemed like it came out of a movie—sitting tall in a wheelchair next to the window, the sunlight gently falling on her through the glass. Opening with a humorous story, she soon turned serious and told her family that the time had come for her to prepare them for life without her. In turn, her family respected her wishes. There was prayer, and there was song—equal parts sorrowful as joyful. In every moment, we were surrounded by her parting message—that even when she was gone, her family and the love that bound them would remain. By the end, there was not a dry eye in the room.

In the days that followed, Grace's hospital room came into bloom, filled with fresh flowers of every color and variety. Amidst beauty that was no less exquisite for its ephemerality, I poured her beetroot juice and listened to her plans. Her deepest-held wish to cook for her family for Thanksgiving. Her Bible to her sister, her earrings to her niece, this ring to her adopted niece. Her desire to have her body cremated, so that her ashes could be spread over the water to become a part of the Earth. Through these conversations I came to admire how this self-possessed woman gracefully accepted her own mortality and generously sent her energy outwards, instead of inwards.

A few days later, I found myself on the receiving end of critical feedback. Grace's room had become a calm oasis in the hospital for me, and I found myself rushing there and crying, "Will I ever become a good doctor?" She comforted me with the certainty and gravity hard-won from lived experience, telling me "Some days are tough, but you've come too far."

When I met Grace, I was a fearful, striving medical student—but she reaffirmed to me that try as the training process might, it could not strip away my humanity and strength. When I think of her, I promise to myself despite the challenges to continue practicing medicine with the same purpose as when I first began—to take a genuine interest in the lives of other people, to assist others with their health so that they in turn can accomplish their goals, to send my energy outwards.

SUMMER CROCODILES

Community health fairs are one of my favorite ways to engage with the community and practice my communication skills. It's also a nice break from rotating between our usual 12 standardized patients in our stuffy clinical skills lab.

It was a hot summer day and some students and I were operating a station that provided free blood pressure readings to fair attendees. By the time we organized the blood pressure cuffs and displayed a colorful array of flyers on our table, people started rolling in.

A man in his early 50's came up to me - my first patient. After greeting him, chatting a bit, and listening for Korotkoff sounds, I let him know his results. "Okay, so I measured your blood pressure to be 140/80. It's a bit high, so you should follow up with your primary doctor so it can be repeated."

"Oh and what does that number mean?" he asked.

Proud that I was prepared for this moment, I handed him one of our flyers with the American Heart Association's BP classifications. The man looked at me and said "Yeah, but can you tell me what this means" as he pointed to a greater-than sign on the flyer.

Pause.

I quickly had to dig through my brain spaces and recall my second-grade arithmetic to try to explain this symbol as clear as possible.
First Aid didn't prepare me for this.

"So this is the greater-than sign. It means that the number before it is greater than the one after," I said.

"But what about it over here, that number is smaller," He replied.

"Well, that one is the less-than sign. It's the same symbol but flipped."

"Oh."

"Imagine the symbol is like a crocodile. The crocodile always wants to eat the larger number." I did my best at remaining calm and collected because I knew the importance of non-judgmental patient interactions. The underclassmen were looking up to me in shock as I finessed this interaction.

The man was scribbling notes on the back of the AHA handout. It was clear that he was determined to learn. For the next 10 minutes, I sat with him explaining the symbols and the different BP classifications. He was so grateful. He told me no one has ever explained this stuff to him before.

Wow.

I always thought that as a student, my voice didn't have much of an impact on the patient experience, but I guess sometimes it's the simplest things that mean the most. I hope my crocodiles follow him for years to come.

GOING WHERE NO ONE HAS GONE BEFORE

It is hard to even dream or imagine that I am sitting in a medical school lecture hall training to be a physician. I am feeling the heart racing, exhilarating rush of taking patient histories and attempting to perform physical exams. I am learning from a beautiful woman who decided to donate her body, so that students like me could become educated well-informed physicians.

I wonder why is it so hard for me to believe that I am sitting here in this seat? I took all of the pre-med classes and studied for the MCAT until my brain throbbed with fatigue just like any other "gunning" future physician. But unlike many students who enter medical school, I did not have any contacts to medicine growing up. I did not have a friendly neighbor doctor, friends who were physicians, or any family who had ventured to trek the path that I had set out on.

It can be astonishingly lonely to feel like you are the sole supporter of your dreams. To feel that you are going somewhere that no one else you know has gone. To add to these feelings of isolation, I am biracial and from the Deep South, meaning I have faced my fair share of implicit and explicit bias. I have seen the shocked look on teacher's faces when they realize that I am smarter than they perceive me to be because of my appearance.

I am so proud to be in medical school and to have faced my fears, deciding to go where no one has gone before. I have met amazing physicians and classmates who make me feel like I am a part of a prestigious group. I do not feel that same loneliness and isolation. I am no longer "going in it alone," and I am well on my way to being an accepting, compassionate physician.

I strive to make it as a physician, so that up and coming future physicians can look to me and know that someone like them has beat the odds. I am so thankful to be going where no one else has gone!

RAY OF SUNSHINE

Given that I'm prone to vaso vagaling out (yes, I'm *that* med student), I knew I had to prepare for my first day of neurosurgery rotation. 16 ounces of water, 8 hours of sleep, and 1 hastily prepared bowl of oatmeal later, I was ready to go.

After morning rounds, I changed into my scrubs, wrote my name on the OR white board, and pulled my sterile gown and gloves, internally patting myself on the back that I didn't accidentally bump into any of the already prepared sterile fields.

In comes the attending neurosurgeon and with a smile on my face, I nervously stammer out, "Hi, I'm the third year medical student who will be rotating with you for the next month." Without looking up at me, he replies, "Oh, so you're my dark cloud for the month?"

Like most med students in this situation, I internally panic as my thoughts scatter in about a billion directions, similar to what I imagine a galaxy imploding on itself to look like. "Is that a rhetorical question or do I actually try to answer it," I think. Not being able to form fully cohesive thoughts, I blurt out, "Black cloud or ray of sunshine, I guess it depends on how you look at it."

"Great, not only have I embarrassed myself, but I bet he will put that I defy authority on my evals now," I reflect. To my surprise though, barely perceptible, I see the corners of his mouth turn up into a small secret smile. "Surgeon myth #1 has officially been disproven, surgeons do smile," I take note. "Perhaps this first day won't turn out to be the crashing trainwreck I thought it was going to be."

A MONTHLY PHENOMENON

A wellness visit with a teenage female wraps up.
Everything looks normal.

"Is there anything else you would like to discuss today?"
"I want something to stop my bleeding each month."
"Can you tell me a little more about that concern?"

With tears in her eyes she says, "I want something to
make me stop bleeding each month – I can't keep losing
my babies."

After a full workup, it was determined that the patient
believed that her monthly menstrual cycle was a series of
miscarriages. At a young age, she dropped out of school
to farm and help provide for her family, so she was never
taught about her body or what the menstrual cycle was.

Each time she bled, she thought she lost another baby. I
felt heartbroken; I can't imagine the sorrow, pain and
confusion she felt monthly, thinking she lost another
child.

Lack of education about something that is so common
and natural as a menstrual cycle caused devastating
monthly pain that put this patient under immense stress.
While it can sometimes feel like a battle against the clock
to finish patient visits in 15 minutes, there has to be
space and time provided to assess patient's
understanding of their own body and medical
knowledge. There were so many missed opportunities in
her past medical visits where she could have been taught
about this natural process. We can never assume; we
must always ask and educate our patients. I reflect on
this story when I feel overwhelmed, to remind myself of
the privilege we have of being our patients' teachers.

MORE THAN MEETS THE EYE

After waiting for an hour to get my admission during one of my evening shifts, I finally got the text from my resident. She gave me 2 facts about my patient: his name and age. Don't know why he's here, don't know anything else about him. I walk in and start with my profound question, "So...what brings you in today?"

Through my history and physical, I learned that he had intractable vomiting for 6 days, 7-8 times a day, including 2-3 times throughout the night. He obviously had not been able to eat, sleep, let alone rest peacefully. His labs came out and he was positive for hepatitis A infection. And as I ran down my list of questions about risk factors for viral hepatitis A, I learned about his sexual activities. He admitted to having had sex with at least 10-11 women within the past 2 months, some who he found online. He was married and had 3 kids.

My first thought was, "Wow, what was he thinking? What is going on in his family?" Sexual history is already a sensitive topic, and I could have easily just assumed he is the "type of person" to sleep around casually. But I was unconvinced. I sat down next to him and started asking about his relationship with his wife – how he is doing emotionally. He then told me that about 7-8 months ago, he witnessed his wife sleeping with another man in his house.

My entire viewpoint was put into question. How traumatic would that be to see the love of your life in bed with another stranger? Who wouldn't be affected after seeing that? The unbounded sexual behavior that seemed incredibly irresponsible before seemed almost .... understandable? I was not there to place judgement on his actions, and I was grateful that my patient was open enough to tell me about this event that must have been very traumatic for him.

This conversation built the trust between me and my patient that carried us throughout the rest of his stay. By the time he was being discharged, he said to me, "Thank you for being so kind to me and taking care of me. You saved my life. I feel so blessed. Thank you."

I hope he knows how much he taught me, too.

GIVING SOME MORE

"The joy is in the giving, so when the joy is gone, when the giving starts to feel more like a burden, that's when you stop. But if you're like most people I know, you give till it hurts, and then you give some more."

This quote is from Grey's Anatomy. The fictional characters inspired me. I even quoted the show on my personal statement to land a spot in medical school. Old habits die hard, huh?

I was sandwiched between long-legged classmates when my mind drifted back to this quote. The hematologist oncologist took me there. Why was the doctor who turned patient in his own field not jaded or angry? He motioned to us with body language that demanded my attention. You enter every patient room with your head and your heart. Every single time.

I had a visceral reaction. How can we give when we are constantly being depleted?

School needs me. Family needs me. I definitely need the gym. But after I call a friend in a different time zone, because she needs me too. I'll call before I prep for PBL. But that has to go before I call mom, because she's a 15-minute talker instead of the 30 seconds my dad takes to make sure I am still breathing.

My hand shot up. "Have you ever experienced entering a patient room with just your head to protect your heart?" Because at some point, the giving becomes a burden. And it only makes sense to stop there, right?

Yes. But mostly a resounding no.

The stoic cardiothoracic surgeon used to keep patients with acute aortic dissection at arm's length. Why give your heart to someone that could die on your operating table in the following 10 minutes?

But then he told us about how he replaced self-preservation with a ritual. He watched planes take off and named the patients he lost. A personal and painful goodbye, but he did it anyway.

I wish I could say that the epiphany that followed was filled with rising butterflies. But it wasn't. To be honest, I am still sorting out my feelings. I think there are going to be days that I am able to give it all. But there are going to be days that a patient's prognosis will tempt me to go heavy on the medical knowledge and light on the emotional empathy. The latter scares me.

I walked away from that panel realizing that I am in the business of giving till it hurts, then giving some more. And for some reason even with my fears laid out on this page, it doesn't seem too bad.

A NEW NORMAL

The hospital was different than before. It looked the same, with the same sunlit hallways, the same sterile floors. Walking through the hospital, you might not notice anything had changed. That is, until you realized you were walking alone. In these COVID-19 times, restrictions have been placed on who can enter the hospital. Stickers dictating a 6-foot distance between people cover the floors. I still see employees moving through the halls, following routine in a new normal.

I thought I would be nervous interviewing my first patient, but I felt oddly safe behind my face mask, face shield and glasses, and with 6 feet between us. No one could see my confusion, surprise or uncertainty. The silences could pass as thoughtful pauses. There is safety in this newfound anonymity.

This ambiguity goes both ways, however. With the masks, you can only really see what is strong enough to reach someone's eyes, but are those eyes squinting from a smile or contempt? Is that an eye roll, or is it just uncomfortably hot under the mask? It's hard to read someone's face when most of it is covered. It's hard to make a connection. There are no more smiles, no comforting taps on the shoulder when someone breaks down. I find myself using exaggerated expressions with patients, hoping the expressions somehow reach my eyes. I hope they feel less lonely, but the honest truth is, I'm not sure.

"I can't watch the news anymore without crying," she says, looking to the ceiling in an attempt to dry her eyes. "People are dying without their loved ones." This comes from one of our patients, who hasn't seen her husband in weeks. With COVID-19, there are new, painful limitations. Family meetings are often done over Zoom, and visitations are limited to extreme situations. The new normal is difficult for care providers, but it doesn't hold a candle to how it is for our patients.

Many of our patients are lonely and homesick. They're without their greatest sources of support at their time of greatest need. As a student, I know I won't be the one to solve anyone's medical problem. I wasn't sure what my role would look like in this strange COVID-19 world. After a week in the hospital, one of our most important goals as medical students has become clear — in this new, isolated normal, we have to find different ways in which we can connect and be there for our patients.

What does that look like? To give you the classic med student answer, I'm not sure, but I'll find out for you.

HONORS DURING CORONA

I had heard about coronavirus once prior to the COVID-19 pandemic. I was studying for Step 1 and was watching SketchyMicro – the infamous medical student cartoon study aid. The sketch "Kingdom of SARS" opened with the narrator saying "Coronavirus, it's not a super high yield virus." If only the creators knew that this non-high yield virus would end up changing the world.

In late February, after the Biogen outbreak in Boston, local hospitals diligently prepared for patients and everyone's anxiety levels skyrocketed. As an MS3 on the Infectious Disease service, I was terrified. The only things I knew about coronavirus came from that Sketchy video and a few articles I had read. I had heard that people were dying and grew fearful because I now found myself on the front lines of this disease.

After a stressful week on the ID service, I made it to my last day and was ready to leave when my attending asked if I wanted to see one last consult. I obliged and went to see a patient with suspected aspiration pneumonia. We spent about 30 minutes together with his family and towards the end of the visit, the patient's daughter asked whether he could have coronavirus. She and her daughters had just arrived from China a couple weeks ago and then her father became ill. It was in this moment that I felt my stomach in my throat. I thought to myself, "Did I just expose myself to coronavirus because I wanted to suck up to my attending?" My attending reassured everyone that this was an unlikely scenario. However, I couldn't get the fear out of my mind. We left the patient's room, discussed the case, and I left the hospital.

On my way home, I received a call from my senior resident. He informed me that the patient I had just seen was being tested for COVID-19 and that I needed to immediately go home and self-quarantine until his results returned. I stayed home googling coronavirus for five days until I finally received the good news that the patient had not tested positive. My experience made me realize that so many patients feel this way every time they're awaiting a test result. They're scared, curious, and anxious, and we as healthcare providers often forget to acknowledge this uncertainty. Although I wish I had never experienced this scare, I feel that I'm now able to better empathize with my patients. Hopefully, by being able to validate their feelings, I will be able to gain their trust in not only the healthcare field but in me as their future physician.

PLEASE, GET THE BIOPSY

The doctor pulled up our next patient's CT scan and pointed out the spot on her lung that he suspected was cancer. We went into the patient's room to talk about the findings, but to my surprise, her response was of anger instead of worry. She refused a biopsy.

I think my mouth dropped open right then and there! I couldn't believe she was refusing to have this procedure. If this was cancer, it may have been caught early enough to be treated; this didn't have to be a death sentence... if only she'd let us biopsy it to find out!

I didn't sleep that night, I felt like crying, and I did. It was too close to a reminder of my situation. My father was diagnosed years earlier with pancreatic cancer, but it was not caught in time and his PET scan was described as a "starry night sky." How was this patient refusing to let us help her? What if this could be treated and she could live another 20 years? What if she kept refusing the biopsy and only when it became too late wanted help? My mind never paused for a second that night.

As much as I wanted to call this patient on a daily basis and beg her to get the biopsy, I had to push her to the back of my mind and focus on our other patients. I'm learning the hard way- if the patient doesn't want to help themselves, there's much less we can do.

A few weeks later, I ran into the pulmonologist I was working with previously. Of course, I had not forgotten about our patient with the ominous spot on her lung, and she was the first thing I asked him about. He smiled and told me, "I was able to convince her after all to get the biopsy." I didn't think twice about asking for the results, that was enough.

THE PATIENT THAT GOT AWAY

It was 6:42 PM. I was near the end of my shift when the ED called. A 55-year-old male with 10/10 chest pain was being admitted to our team. Being the eager medical student, I finish chart reviewing, call the patient from the ED waiting room, and begin the interview.

"Finally! I've been sitting for over 12 hours. Am I finally getting a bed and IV pain medications?"

"Uhh...not yet sir. I apologize but we're still waiting for a bed to open up. In the meantime, I'm a 3rd year medical student from the admitting team. It's nice to meet you. What brings you to the hospital today?"

"I've told my story to two other physicians already! I'm not answering these questions again. Are you giving me a bed or not?"

I reply that he will receive a bed as soon as one opens up. My resident joins me mid-interview reiterating the same thing. I nervously continue the interview, hoping the patient will start answering my questions. But before I knew it the patient was out his chair, asking the ER staff for the nearest hospital. Soon after, he was gone AMA.

What just happened? How did I botch the interview so badly that made the patient leave AMA?

I walked back to the team room in shame, expecting the worst. But as soon as I walked in, my senior said, "Way to go, you guys! That's one less patient for us which means we get to go home on time." I was stunned. My initial thought of the situation was that I was a complete failure, yet my senior was giving me praise. I quickly ignored my own feelings of inadequacy and cherished the compliment, thinking this situation would help my evaluations.

Two days later, I attended a process group. I was paired with an attending who helped me process the situation. Before I knew it, I was crying, tears streaming down my face. When did my priorities change that I valued the praise of my senior over the well-being of a patient? What happened throughout medical school that made me lose so much of the empathy and compassion that I started with?

Luckily for me, the attending reminded me that it wasn't too late to change. Recognizing this issue was a major accomplishment but redefining my practice of medicine was the necessary change. To this day, I strive to treat all patients with empathy and compassion, which is to understand their situation fully and to advocate for their needs incessantly. Whenever I encounter a difficult situation, I will always think back to this experience and never forget about the patient that got away.

ELSA'S HAIR

On my pediatrics rotations, my first patient arrived on the same day that I started my month on the oncology service. She was an energetic little blonde 4-year-old girl who reminded me of myself at that age.

Sadly, she was on our service to be worked up for a suspicious lung mass found when evaluating her for asthma. As time progressed, we learned that she had a rare pediatric tumor that was part of an inherited cancer syndrome. This meant that even if she survived this cancer, she would likely develop an additional one or more cancer elsewhere when she was in adolescence or early adulthood. I read case reports and researched the literature for any hope. This was my 3rd clinical rotation and I could not let my first pediatric patient down. I memorized all the information I could on the pathology, clinical course, and prognosis.

Accompanying my attending to deliver the diagnosis, I carefully listened to him deliver this earth-shattering news. I watched the family's heart break before my eyes as the mother searched for words and attempted to catch her breath between tears. Their other two children would need to be tested as well.

What came next was clear. This patient and her family did not need the pathophysiology or research I had done. Rather, they needed support.

From then on, that is what I became. Every afternoon I would go back to visit this patient and I would play the Frozen sound track on my phone and braid her hair like Elsa's from the Disney movie, play with her "Shopkins dolls," or speak with her mother about how she is doing. I connected the mother with social work to get more family and medical leave time. But mostly, I was present and listened.

For rounds one Saturday, I wore my hair like Elsa and I will never forget the way her little face lit up when she saw me. This patient will always have a special place in my heart.

She taught me that medicine is much more than being competent and knowing the cutting-edge research, but the practice of medicine is all encompassing, and we need to make a commitment to provide genuine, patient-centered compassionate care.

THE WEARY TRAVELER

The music drifted softly through the air when I saw her small body in the hospice bed. As the nurse turned down the soothing melody that played in the room, I caught a bit of the chorus, "hello, hello...goodbye, goodbye." I was taken aback by how fitting the chorus was. It had only been twenty minutes since I had last walked into C.G.'s room. Now however, her soft, frail body looked strangely different. C.G had passed. My partners and I helped change her sheets and prepare her for the funeral home that would be coming later. We tried to work quickly enough so her son, who had stepped outside to call family, could spend time with her. The nurse opened the window. She told us that this was her way of ensuring the soul was not trapped in the hospice and could move on.

This strange place where spirituality and science met greatly intrigued me. There was a comforting rhythm behind the care of patients in the hospice inpatient floor. It did not have the cold, sterile, and clinical feel of a hospital. The entire staff spoke in voices like leather, strong enough to carry the burden of bad news, but soft enough to convey it. The warmth in each room made me reflect on the history of hospice. First originated in England, its purpose was to give refuge to weary travelers. It seemed that even in modern times, the meaning of hospice had not really changed. There were many illnesses, such as cancer and Alzheimer's, that robbed patients of their independence and even their identity. Each person that came to the hospice was a traveler on their own journey of life. Some had grown weary from a slew of grueling treatments. Some wanted to spend the time they had left with family while still feeling like themselves.

Despite the circumstances, the welcoming and comforting environment of hospice reflected the way in which healthcare professionals interacted with each other. The fluidity in the communication and the subsequent course of action made me feel a sense of belonging. As I observed how the staff worked together, I felt an immense sense of wonder. I can think of nothing more rewarding than helping someone navigate the certainty in morality and the uncertainties of what comes after death. Regardless of which specialty I pursue, I will encounter many weary travelers. Traveling life's path is difficult. However, I have learned that something as simple as a gentle squeeze of a hand can make the journey a little easier.

WASICU WITH SCABIES

Scabies. I had them. I was in Guatemala just months before, and the pattern they created on my skin was all too familiar; their characteristic tunneling forming burrows under my skin on my arms, chest, groin, and neck. I must have shared a bunk bed with them last night, and they had freeloaded on my skin without my permission. I needed to give myself a thorough permethrin bath, and ASAP.

I was inside the Indian Reservation, and the only nearby pharmacy was associated with the Indian Health Service (IHS), which I could not use because I was not part of the Lakota tribe. I am Wašíču*. Yet, I quickly realized that my current lack of pharmacy was a small inconvenience in comparison to the challenges faced by those from this and many other American Indian communities. So many of my patients face similar difficulties when accessing healthcare. Many have food, transportation, and housing insecurities. Nothing is easy to access.

I drove to a pharmacy in Nebraska. Upon returning to the bunkhouse that was provided to us during our cultural immersion week, I took the most thorough shower of my life! Later that day, I rejoined my team to continue exploring the many factors that affect the Lakota community in order to help me better treat all our American Indian patients. I still may have been itchy, but the memory of scabies paled in comparison to the lessons I learned.

*Wašíču: 1. of European descent 2. white immigrants (now descendants of) who migrated west and conquered this land "stealing all the fat."

FAILING

I didn't pass. Suddenly it felt like bricks were tumbling from the sky. The shadow of imposter syndrome, ever present but previously reduced to a lazy wisp, instantaneously grew and enveloped me whole. On an average Tuesday after morning report, I had been called by the school registrar and told that I hadn't passed the pediatric shelf exam. Instead of the fifth percentile required to pass the clerkship, I had made ... fourth.

How did this happen? Reasons raced through my mind. It was my first rotation. I was burned out from studying for STEP1. I was more concerned with adjusting to hospital and faculty expectations. They put me in the Pediatric ICU the very week of my exam and I came home after hours and crying every day... Bah. Excuses.

The rest of the morning was miserable. I was on my OB/GYN clerkship and people caught me in the side hall reeling from the news: exhaustion and feelings of shame and uncertainty sinking in. It might seem silly to see someone crying about a test: indeed, there are so many more things worth crying about—in a hospital, of all places. Still, never before had I failed such an important exam or class. Kind residents found me and were compassionate: "It happens. It's fine. I know someone who didn't even pass STEP1 and is now head of Anesthesia..." Their intentions comforted me for a second but then slid off amidst old insecurities creeping up. I felt like I had let not only myself down, but also my family rooting for me on the other side of the country, my brother looking up to me, and my classmates who always gave me the benefit of the doubt and assumed I was smarter than I really was. I was sent to a call room to collect myself for however long I needed and hid from my classmates for much of the day. For the rest of the year, I was too embarrassed to talk about failing, but urged everyone I saw: Study for Peds. It's REALLY hard.

I passed on my second try months later. We don't often talk about or take seriously the struggles and failures along the way in med school. There's the feeling of: if I can't handle this much, how can I be trusted with patients? My classmates are so smart and don't have problems with school, so I've got to be able to catch up. But those thoughts contributed to me feeling alone and behind. The following year, I broke my silence to the rising MS3's. Proudly telling them I had failed and made it back was important to me to share.

You never know who might need to hear it.

SYMBRACHYDACTYLY

At the first week of orientation, I was excited. But also, nervous.

I was nervous that someone would realize I did not belong and that they made a mistake. That nagging feeling persisted even a couple weeks after school started, until I realized no one was going to change their mind. Not even when I asked for accommodations.

I was born with symbrachydactyly. I am used to doing things a little differently, whether it's opening a jar or tying my hair. Medical school would be no exception. While I was confident in my academic ability and my ability to engage with patients, I was worried about my ability to perform manual tasks, such as physical exams. Physical exams are essential – it's how we are able to determine what symptoms patients may be feeling and how we may be able to resolve them.

When I realized there were "concrete ways" students were expected to perform physical exams, I met with the program coordinator and physician who ran the clinical skills program. Although I discussed having a disability in my application to medical school, I did not know who in the school knew I had a disability. One of the individuals I met with asked me if I was confident in my ability to do everything that was required. It was a hard question to answer because I did not know any of the exams by heart; I have never even performed any of the exams on a person. How am I supposed to confidently tell you I can do everything if I do not know what everything entails? My response was that I have confidence in my ability to be flexible and adapt. Because I have been doing that my whole life.

I would say one of the most challenging parts of medical school for me is being in a lecture and hearing a faculty member say "with both hands." I would ask, after class and before seeing the standardized patient, why the exam had to be done that way. I ask because sometimes we are so stuck on how we traditionally do things that we assume there is the only one correct method.

Students with disabilities are present, including in medicine, but I felt alone on my journey. I am lucky to have been connected to a student ahead of me in medical school who wears a prosthetic and knows which design works best for them as they practice medicine. As I have their guidance and the knowledge that a person without a hand can expertly practice medicine, I have become more secure in my place in my program and more confident in my ability to become a great physician.

DEDICATED

I'm thinking of how I got here. Four years of college. Four waitlists. Four acceptances. Two years of medical school.

I'm thinking of how I got here, and I don't want to waste it. Potential is a terrible thing to waste. And I'm wondering why human beings can get so close, their goals palpable, yet feel so tired. Scared of squandering their entire journey, but unable to find the flicker of motivation to ignite them.

I asked myself a lot this year how gratitude could become so mixed with depression. How blessings could line my bedroom, my car, my bound books, the hugs from friends, and yet I could still feel so alone.

Some of our blessings are handed to us on a silver platter. My silver platter is Algerian. It is my mother staying up waiting for me to get home. It is my mother brewing mint tea with my "hold the green tea this time mom, it's really late." It is my mother dropping off food on finals week, picking up my calls when I cry, when I laugh, when I just want to talk.

Some of our blessings are earned to us through sweat and tears, handed to us like a well-deserved diploma. My diploma is medical school. My diploma is getting rejected once, then applying again anyways. My diploma is spending hours of my honeymoon writing admission essays instead of exploring a new city. My diploma is making it, and still feeling like I may not belong. My diploma is staying anyways.

And this is what we do. We plan, we wait, we reach our goal. Maybe we don't, so we find a new one. Little time to pause, reflect, then quickly turn around.

I have thought of Step 1 for years. Years have come, passed, and in two weeks, I start dedicated. And I think of the first person who called it "dedicated," and all the words that make it so: loyalty, integrity, investment, devotion. And I think of all the words I have been thinking of instead: fear of failure, anxiety, stress, loss of time.

I'm thinking again of how I got here. And how where I want to go is not a place. I will not "arrive" at what I want for this exam. There is no way to "get there." I will have to strive for it, create it in small, impactful ways. I will need my silver platters and my diplomas. And have to redefine what it means for me to be "dedicated."

A CONSTANT CYCLE

Today, a practice exam told me I was wrong 18 out of 40 times. Yes, it stung a little. I marked one incorrect because I couldn't remember the name of vitamin B12. Another I read too quickly and mistook schistocytes for schistosomiasis. One I had not heard of half the potential answers and spent a long timing reviewing the correct explanation to learn something completely new. Question and answer, confirm and relearn. It's a constant cycle.

And it's such a strange cycle we med students go through. Always learning, but never knowing quite enough. Being told we're wrong, inexperienced, naïve. Patients looking for the real doc in the room. Residents chuckling at our silly mistakes, broad differentials, and zebra diagnoses no one has seen in clinic for 30 years. Learning from mistakes, then making new ones. It's a constant cycle.

Do we ever get to the point where we know things? A time where we feel comfortable and certain, full of confidence that we're not faking? This seems unattainable and so far away.

Applying to med school was the most stressful process I had ever experienced. A real make or break moment. Now matching to my dream residency holds that place. Then it will be fellowship, then job placement. It never ends. There is always something next, just out of reach. It's a constant cycle.

Then, 1 month, 1 year, 4 years go by in this cycle!

We don't notice, but day by day we make progress. When did I start to get better at answering questions? Did I hack the system? Did rote memorization finally work? Or possibly, could it really be, I was learning exactly the way my mentors said I would? My notes improved and were praised by my attending, presentations became clearer and focused, and relationships with patients strengthened. I present my findings, thoughts, and recommendations to the resident without stuttering or forgetting something and having to recheck. Unaware of these small improvements being made, I didn't notice how I began to embrace this constant cycle.

Progress is made and seemingly unattainable goals are reached. It doesn't happen in an instant or without a lot of hard work. But it happens. We cycle through and we prevail. We learn and grow stronger. We aren't stuck in a constant cycle; we're taking control of it. We're expanding it and pushing it to its max. Day by day, practice question by practice question, patient by patient, we go. We run that cycle and then we run it some more.

MAKINGS OF A MED STUDENT

I have this patient. It's been over a week and everything keeps getting worse. He is a sweet older gentleman with end stage lung cancer who came in with difficulty breathing. I thought I would find out he had died when I came back a couple of days ago, but he felt better over the weekend and was able to visit with his family.

When he returned, he deteriorated rapidly. We could do nothing more. The family decided on home hospice the next morning.

Yesterday, when I came in, I saw that he was still on our service. My resident pulled me off his case because there was nothing more the team was doing for him. It wasn't a learning experience for me anymore. I got a different patient that he thought would be more worth my time.

I went to see him anyway. When I walked in the room, my heart broke. His wife was sitting next to the bed, holding his hand. She looked as if she had been crying and hadn't slept much. And my patient. I don't think he noticed that his wife was there next to him.

Seeing him, I didn't think he would make it to the end of the day, let alone make it home. I realized then how completely out of my element I was. What could I possibly contribute to this situation? Standing there, I had no idea.

I was at a loss for words and the only thing I could think to say was, "Is there anything I can do for you?" His wife, slightly taken aback by my obviously futile question, said we could pray for them. We prayed together right there. It was unlike anything I've ever experienced. I don't know how to describe it. It felt like for the first time in my medical school career I had actually done something that mattered.

He died the next day. He was my last patient on my Medicine rotation. As I sat taking the Shelf exam, I thought about those last moments of his life. Then I thought about all of the things I'm required to do as a student – exams, lectures, answering questions, writing notes, and filling out countless surveys and feedback forms. I used to think that these things were what helped turn a student into a physician. Walking through those last moments with that family reminded me that the tasks of medical school are not an end in and of themselves. They are a set of tools that give me the opportunity to engage compassionately in the lives of patients and their families. The tools are necessary in quality physicians, but they're really just the beginning.

ORATOR IN TRAINING

In society, we talk about "medicalization"- the act of coming to define traits, processes, or events as medical conditions. This implies there is a treatment, though that's not always true. To me, the process of becoming a doctor seems itself to be a medicalization of the self – one in which we do not have the pathology, and yet it becomes a part of us. Not only from our understanding of disease or how hospitals operate, but also in the ways we communicate and frame our thinking.

I was giving a presentation at the end of my Internal Medicine clerkship with some of the phrases I've come to rely on. I eventually stopped to think, "Wow, I'm starting to sound like a doctor." But there was a moment of hesitation where I wasn't sure that was a good thing. Phrases as seemingly non-medical as "lower on my differential" or "negative work up" sound like they could be understood by anyone. Or do they?

I feel as though I've lost sight of what words are part of normal human vernacular, and which have simply become a part of mine as a result of this training process. And I'm only two years into training - what will I sound like by the end? Such phrases, along with the more physiological ones like "acute on chronic" or "poor substrate" act as flags that assign meaning. The signposts are important for communicating ideas that often exist in persistently gray territory, but they are part of an acquired script nonetheless.

Vocabulary is part of the medicalization, but there is also a specific cadence that surfaces. Last year, a preceptor warned me that there's a certain lilt that residents acquire as they train – one she warned me to avoid falling into. "It makes them sound like they're bored," she said. At the time, I had no idea what she was talking about, but I was determined to pay attention. A few months into rotations, and now I know exactly the tone. No one means to sound bored, but we adopt the behaviors and rules around us, especially when we are surrounded by people to whom we look as role models and teachers.

This week, toward the end of my clerkship, I heard another student give a presentation. For the first time, he had a new tone. He had The Lilt. Will it happen to me? As I learn to inhabit my role in the medical world, I hope I don't lose the other aspects of my language - the tones and references that have been shaped by history, literature, family - the ones that make the me who is more than just a med student.

WHERE THE LIVING LEARN FROM THE DEAD

Above the entrance into anatomy lab is a quote I have learned by heart: "Where the living learn from the dead."

I vaguely remember a quick powerpoint introducing dissections and telling us how to prepare at the end of a 3-hour class. Yet, the feeling when our small groups finally arrived at the lab was simply indescribable.

Bright eyed and naïve, we had received scrubs, tools and dissectors. But amongst the chaos of medical school, we didn't have time to really think about the impact of what we would soon be doing.

On January 3rd, around lunch time, we marched towards the anatomy changing rooms, the smell of formaldehyde permeating the walls. I took refuge in the bathroom to gather my thoughts and make sure my hair was pulled back. I walked under that quote for the first time, barely reading the words, yet memorizing them somehow. Clusters of students walked in, progressively getting quieter as we walked through to the last room assigned to us. Slightly unsteady on my feet in my hospital clogs, I joined my groupmates around table 15.

He was facing down the first time I saw him. Maybe that helped. The next time he was laying up. We saw his face and read his card: male, 51, #####, hanging.

Grouped around him in an oddly solemn silence among the discussions, we stood for a little while. I went home that day, my thoughts running wild. Was I sad? Was I thankful? Was I ashamed for not crying? Was I afraid? I kept thinking that could have been me, that could even still be me one day. Would I ever do that? Why did he choose it?

Then I held his hand. Everything became so much clearer. I held his hand as my scalpel, forceps, scissors, and fingers explored his axilla. I held on tighter as the brachial plexus became visible. There was a reason he decided this. The best thanks I can ever give is to become a good doctor. There will be days when I am sad and have trouble cutting, and days I feel guilty and selfish for not being sad. Those days will always exist but because of him I will remember I can have mixed feelings. I may never know his name or his story, but he will always be with me.

Somehow, I will make him proud.

THINGS WE CAN'T FIX

"Sit behind me, your back against the wall, and remember not to look him in the eye."

Of all the doctors I've had the opportunity to shadow, Dr. Silver serves not solely as a medical doctor, but as a gatekeeper, assisting his patients in battling their inner demons. As I walked into the exam room to observe my first case of antisocial personality disorder, I approached it with a voyeuristic blend of curiosity and trepidation, fascinated by the destructive potential of an individual with psychopathy. Our paths appeared to be diametrically opposed. While I sat in Dr. Silver's office to fulfill my dreams and desires, Mr. X was presently seeking help just to make it through his day.

By the time I entered the exam room, Mr. X had pillaged the cabinets, and began to take aim at Dr. Silver and myself with a reflex hammer. Though his behaviors were meant to intimidate, it was impossible to ignore palpable waves of anguish he was feeling. Although he had a lack of empathy, Mr. X was lonely, having alienated friends and family. The climate of suffering Mr. X lived in led to anxiety, depression, and suicidal ideation. He refused to be treated by anyone other than Dr. Silver, threatening homicide for all psychiatrists who attempted to aid him. Even after years of sessions, there would be no healing, only antipsychotics as the proxy for glue in the cracks of his broken moral compass.

From my clinical exposure, I've seen a little bit of a lot. Whether a client has a Chiari malformation or angioedema, every patient requires reassuring confidence and warmth, conveyed through a physician's bedside manner. While one's physical body is important in life, and the preservation of its health is paramount, I regard Dr. Silver's emotional ministering to be just as vital. His sensitivity toward a man whose dominant force in life was resistance to authority was astounding, something I hope to replicate in the future. This was the moment at which the lifelong ambition to become a physician was solidified. On this day, Dr. Silver's debrief with me focused on how distressing it can seem when there is no cure for what ails a person's mind. The difficulty I will inevitably face in encouraging others to place their trust in me is sometimes daunting, for I will not always be able to fulfill the everyone's needs. Nevertheless, I am eager to make this commitment, for no experiences in my life have been as gratifying as those I have shared intimately with others.

APART

The night I got my white coat, I called you. You said you were proud of me. I'm sorry for all the time we lost.

Daadi, we live a plane-ride, two rickshaws, and a language barrier apart. Even when you lived in America raising me and my brother, I knew so little about you. I knew what I thought were the important things: you were the best at chess in the family, you put a little too much milk in mac and cheese, and you'd always let me have an extra cookie when Ma wasn't looking. And, that you were a doctor. The first doctor I knew in our family—and the only female one. You never said it, but I knew you closed your clinic in India to come take care of me and Vinay.

As I cared for patients, I'd remember how you'd stitch up our cuts, know what meds to give for our stomach aches, and use household herbs to make a paste for burns and rashes. Medicine here is slightly different but so similar. During the long nights when the line patients at the free clinic filled the parking lot, I remember when a neighbor brought her lab results to you for a second opinion: you put on those little circle glasses you'd use to read the Bhagavad Gita. You meant business. I asked how you remembered medicine when you'd closed your clinic years ago. You smiled and said, "medicine and helping are like riding a bike. You don't forget."

After twelve years, when you returned to India, part of me left with you: my Gujarati faded; I forgot parts of the stories you told me at night to help me sleep; I lost the stethoscope you gave me. Our conversations over the phone became the short, empty pleasantries people separated by generations share. I stopped calling every month. I told myself I was busy. I made myself busy because it hurt too much to know how far apart we had drifted.

Despite our distance and fading connection, medicine held us together. Through the years my broken tongue would sketch out what I was feeling, and you immediately knew what I meant—knowing when to console and when to advise. I like to think that even if I will never be able to fully explain to you how much I've wanted to be like you, you know. The distance that separates us shrinks when I'm walking in your footsteps, trying to learn how to ride this bike as well as you still do.

LIKE CHICKEN SOUP

I come from a family of immigrant healthcare professionals. As with any immigrant population, we have brought some of our cultural beliefs and traditions to the new world with us, as bizarre as they may admittedly be considered in our adopted home. My mother is a dentist with a practice in West Hollywood, and my father is an Interventional Cardiologist in South LA. Both completed their higher education in the US and are rational, logical, science-minded people. However, whenever one of us--their children--seemed to be coming down with something, my parents would turn to two remedies first: one alimentary and one spiritual.

The notion of using certain foods to combat illness is cross-cultural; it's just that the types of foods are culturally-specific. For Iranians, chai-ba-nabat (black tea with rock candy) and ash-e-shalgham (turnip stew) are considered the gold standard. Chai is a cure all. Feeling under the weather? Chai. Feeling sad? Chai. Feeling tired? Chai. Sweet tea is considered especially useful if the culprit is thought to be a virus as it helps "flush it out of the system." Growing up, whenever I sensed the aroma of ash-e-shalgham wafting from the kitchen, I knew someone in the house was sick. Much like chicken soup for Westerners, it is THE cold remedy for Iranians in the cold winter months back in the old country. My mother made it with chicken, an assortment of herbs and greens, beans, and of course, giant fleshy turnips.

Another tradition passed down from the days of Zoroastrianism is to burn esfand (wild rue) seeds. The smoke and popping sound from burning the seeds is thought to ward off the "evil eye." My mother would burn the seeds over tin foil on the stove and then circle the foil containing the seeds around our heads three times to keep away bad juju. As an Iranian-American kid trying to fit in with my classmates, traditions like these were the hardest to explain. Having grown up and moved 3000 miles away from home to the Bronx for medical school, I now miss the protective circle of love that the ring of smoke signified.

Reflecting back, these health beliefs seem, at worst, benign, and at best, beneficial. Just the act of having someone care for you in a time of need by making you soup, encouraging you to drink tea, or burning some magical seeds on your behalf, makes you feel cared for and can boost your self-perception of how you feel. Popping a Dayquil or Nyquil just isn't the same.

TELEMEDICINE

Click

Clipboard and laptop in hand, I call in the next patient.
This woman has short hair that looks like it has been
dusted with a salt and pepper shaker - black and white
speckling beginning to show her steadily advancing age.
She carries herself as though hyper-aware of her passing
years; feeling the weight of time on her shoulders,
bleaching her hair and wearing on her skin like
sandpaper pulling down on what was once a young,
crisply carved face. As she seats herself in the cold and
sterile-looking exam room, I notice things seem a bit
asymmetrical about her. The most obvious of which is a
beige compression sleeve on one arm running from her
shoulder to her fingers. I ask why she is wearing it. She
tells me about her radical mastectomy and lymph node
removal. She is here in the office today because she has
lost her ability to feel the touch of her children and
husband on her fingertips and the ground beneath her
toes after the addition of a new chemotherapy drug. The
cancer has taken to her liver and lungs.

Click

I hold my humanity through the screen, dangling by the
thread of my imagination that connects me to her. My
mind filled in these details as I read "68 year-old female
patient presents with metastatic cancer" on my computer
screen, opening my first patient case of the day. I watch
sentences populate the screen as I answer questions
about this distant, unrealized, virtual woman. I actively
fill my thoughts with the sense of her to retain some
semblance of human compassion while I run through
prognostic algorithms in my mind. When this is all over
and she sits in front of me, I hope it will be intact.

LOCKDOWN

Her day starts suddenly, again
like the cracking of an eggshell
There's no going back
to the tranquility just before.

Reality
is harsher than the smell of cauterized flesh
And more stark
than blood on a fresh blouse
Reality has long been a resting place.

Medicine is safer
than those moments between tasks
than these days lacking structure
than the weeks without purpose.

Gone are the days
of struggle with peace
of venture with serenity
Each intellectual pursuit, each insurmountable goal
calms the internal storm
that reality insists on pressurizing.

She can't be alone in this plight
Troubled hearts become lovers
Troubled souls become healers
who aspire to treat all but one
and are damn persistent in that affliction.

The world slows yet the virus spreads
Safe spaces include the home
Safe spaces exclude her home
Medicine missing most poignant
Reality present most unwavering.

Ambition is not lacking
as there is much to still be done
But there is no replacement for medicine
And reality approaches faster
then she could ever run.

A MATTER OF PERSPECTIVE

I know better.
I know nothing, and I am useless.
So don't throw words at me insinuating that
I am knowledgeable.
I know the truth.
Because at the end of each day
I have nothing to contribute to my patients
And I'm not going to dwell on the lie that
I can make a difference in their well-being
Because who am I kidding?
I'm just a med student.
Even though
The patient appreciates my effort
I am still reminded of the fact that
With each suture thrown or dosage drawn
I slow down the resident and the attending
Regardless of whether
I try my best
So
It's hard to believe that
I'm here to learn and grow
Nothing will change the fact that
I think of what lies ahead in the wards as a hindrance
Each morning when
I ask myself
What am I doing here?

(It's easy to think like this when you're feeling DOWN.
But don't forget those days when things are looking UP.
How you read it is all a matter of perspective.)

How sad and bad and mad it was –
But then, how it was sweet!
　　　　　　　　　　– Robert Browning

AFTERWORD

Narrative medicine is a way of thinking about medicine that emphasizes the importance of stories as a crucial component of healthcare. In any healthcare context, one of narrative medicine's most essential questions is,"Who gets to tell the story?" Whose voice is heard, and whose is not? Who is center stage and who is silent?

Historically, patients' voices were often subordinated to those of their physicians. Even today, with enlightened concepts such as shared decision-making and patient-centered medicine receiving well-deserved prominence in healthcare, patients often find it difficult to make themselves heard. They sometimes choose to reclaim their voices through writing first person narratives and poetry, or blogging about their experiences. In this way they are able prioritize their reality by sharing their words with others.

In recent decades, physicians too have realized that they have stories to tell. Just as patients are not simply recipients of healthcare interventions, physicians are not simply automaton delivery systems of such care. Albeit in different ways than patients, physicians too struggle with illness, suffering, and death. They bear the burden holding the lives and wellbeing of other human beings in their hands. They must somehow find that elusive balance between professional and personal commitments. Increasingly, they have turned to writing as a form of self-expression, providing a fascinating and often moving window into their lives. Nurses too, whose bedside experiences is often quite different and more visceral than those of doctors, also choose to share their stories through reflective writing.

And what of medical students? One of the lessons students learn on their Pediatrics rotation in medical school is that children are not "little adults." Similarly, medical students are not "little doctors." Although they do share much in common with physicians, their different developmental stage and level of clinical experience make the experiences of medical students unique. It has been noted that medical students occupy a liminal place in the world of medicine. They are no longer "members of the public," but they are not yet doctors. In this sense, they have a Janus-like quality to them – they still remember the "face" of ordinary people, their humanity; yet they are also learning to adopt the "face" or perhaps the "mask" of the physician. This unique perspective gives them an understanding of medicine that cannot be obtained in any other way.

Yet it is not always an easy thing for students to find and express their authentic voices. Many students have commented that too often "becoming a physician" seems to involve suppressing or relinquishing core parts of who they are while learning how to develop a medical persona, as the essay "Two Selves" suggests. As is often evident in several of the DOAMS stories, students may suffer from imposter syndrome, the fear that they really do not deserve an opportunity to train as physicians. As a result, they may also worry that their authentic voices somehow "prove" that they don't belong in medicine. In line with this, they are concerned that their physician supervisors may judge them negatively for sharing their reality. Yet they also become aware that this stifling of aspects of self leads to disillusionment, depression, and burn-out. So increasingly medical students take the risk of applying fingers to keyboard to create personal stories that provide distinctive insights into their training experience.

There have been other collections of writings by medical students. What is particularly valuable about Diary of a Medical Student is that the editors have prioritized the emotional journey that occurs during medical training. Of note, they are interested not only in presenting the emotions that medical students undergo, but in excavating the meaning of these emotions. They implicitly ask the question, do the emotions of medical students matter? These essays respond with a resounding yes, showing that it is through awareness of their feelings and their critical reflection on those feelings that doctors become who they will be for the rest of their professional lives.

Wisely, the editors understand that a story does not fully become a story until it is shared, read and reacted to by an engaged reader. Although the title of the collection refers to a "Diary," this is a diary meant to be discovered and read. Of course, the journaling device is in the grand tradition of other literary diaries that always intended an audience (from Anne Frank's Diary of a Young Girl to Virginia Woolf's Diary of a Writer, Che Guevara's and The Absolutely True Diary of a Part-Time Indian [Sherman Alexie]). Such "secret" journals are often radical in content precisely because they are putting forth authentic truth-telling that usually is not meant for public consumption. It is in just such a spirit that Diary of a Medical Student was conceived and executed.

In these "diary entries," medical students recount tales of humor, sorrow, joy and inspiration. These are all commonplace emotional states of course. What is "revolutionary" is that these student-authors claim them proudly and unequivocally. As the Founder's Note suggests, the student-authors are also looking for the meaning behind their emotions; and if there is one overarching meaning they discover, it is their saying, in effect: *Yes, we are human. We embrace the fact that medicine, while often a somber profession, has moments of hilarity and we celebrate these without apology. When patients suffer and die, when we cannot reduce their misery or save their lives, we feel grief, as well as sometimes guilt, frustration, and anger. When a healthy child is born, when a patient and family experience a good death, when a patient recovers, we are happy and feel joy. We are lifted up to be better doctors by the courage of our patients, the sacrifices of our families and the commitment of our role-models.* The emotional reactions to medicine represented in these stories are not the unprofessional responses of naïve beginners, but rather the qualities that will continue to help these students grow into outstanding, compassionate physicians.

In these brief essays, these students are vulnerable, self-deprecating, non-defensive, non-judgmental, compassionate, kind, and humble. They undergo an IV placement to reassure a pediatric patient and risk contracting scabies to put away a homeless patient's meager belongings. They need a hug from a resident. They are willing to laugh at their wardrobe – and diagnostic – mishaps. They accept skepticism and occasional mistrust from patients; and still understand that it is an honor and a privilege to care for all patients, including the disgruntled ones.

The authors of these stories are grateful for their patients' gratitude and discovering that sometimes they can alleviate suffering simply by applying a Band-aid or rubbing someone's hand, praying with them or styling their own hair like that of a pediatric patient's beloved Disney character. They are ready not only to help their patients but to receive wise counsel and guidance from them, the living, the dying, and the dead. Sometimes they simply sit with their dying patients and sometimes they leave when they know they should have stayed. They celebrate their patients as rock stars, are humbled by their courage, and grieve when they pass.

These students take uncomplicated pride when they nail a diagnosis or master a procedure, while learning that they do not need to be perfect, sometimes they will fail, and that sometimes even their physician role models won't have all the answers. In a simple risk of falling test, they find profound lessons about resilience. They are not afraid to feel compassion; and when it doesn't naturally arise, they go in search of it, questioning their assumptions about who is "deserving" of their empathy and who is not. Somehow through clicks of the EMR, telemedicine consults, and the ubiquitous anonymity of pandemic masks and face shields, they make connections with patients.

The student-writers are profoundly aware that medicine suffers from the virus of structural racism as much as the coronavirus and that we must find solutions for both. They know that medicine hurts, but that it is also full of joy. They are brave enough to still ask themselves, "What is truly important to me?" and to live the answer. They hold on to their humanity.

In short, these students are everything we yearn for in our physicians. My fervent hope is that they will continue to be the doctors they already are.

Johanna Shapiro, PhD
Recall Professor, Department of Family Medicine
Director, Program in Medical Humanities & Arts
University of California, Irvine

CONTRIBUTING AUTHORS

It is not lost on us the courage required to craft such personal, honest, and reflective stories for the world to read. We greatly thank each and every one of our contributors for their remarkable work. Without the following medical students, this book would not have been possible.

Aaishwariya Gulani
    University of Central Florida School of Medicine
Abigail E.M. Watson
    Drexel College of Medicine
Ajay N. Sharma
    University of California, Irvine School of Medicine
Alex Wang
    University of California, Irvine School of Medicine
Anabel Starosta
    Harvard Medical School
Anastasiya Haponyuk
    University of New Mexico School of Medicine
Andrea Wakim
    Stritch School of Medicine, Loyola University
Andrew Park
    University of California, San Diego School of Medicine
Angel Reyes
    Harvard Medical School
Austin Buchla
    Tufts University School of Medicine
Avery Olson
    Sanford School of Medicine, University of South Dakota
Brenda T. Wu
    University of California, Davis School of Medicine
Catherine Banh
    University of California, Riverside School of Medicine
Cheyenne Rahimi
    Pacific Northwest University College of Medicine
Christina Grabar
    University of California, Irvine School of Medicine
Christopher Miller
    University of Washington School of Medicine

Daniel Azzam
    University of California, Irvine School of Medicine
David Behrman
    Medical College of Georgia
Diana I. Rapolti
    University of Illinois at Chicago College of Medicine
Donel S. Kelly
    Tufts University School of Medicine
Elizabeth Manuela De Jesus
    Tufts University School of Medicine
Elizabeth Schueth
    Indiana University School of Medicine
Ellery Maya-Altshuler
    University of Florida College of Medicine
Erin Bishop
    The Ohio State University College of Medicine
Gabrielle Cummings
    Mayo Clinic School of Medicine
Galila Flatow
    Albert Einstein College of Medicine
Hannah Shy
    University of Arizona College of Medicine, Tucson
Hayoung Youn
    Lewis Katz School of Medicine, Temple University
Helen Li
    Indiana University School of Medicine
Howard Chang
    Johns Hopkins University School of Medicine
Jacob Stultz
    University of California, San Francisco School of Medicine
Jen Wineke
    Perelman School of Medicine, University of Pennsylvania
Jessica Mgbeojirikwe
    City University of New York School of Medicine
Jo Anderson
    University of Colorado School of Medicine
Joyce L. Zhang
    Drexel University College of Medicine
Juhi Varshney
    University of California, San Francisco School of Medicine
Karlie Snead
    University of Washington College of Medicine
Kevin S. Kang
    Geisel School of Medicine, Dartmouth University

Khodayar Goshtasbi
  University of California, Irvine School of Medicine
Kristin Krumenacker
  Renaissance School of Medicine, Stony Brook University
Lauren Truwit
  Eastern Virginia Medical School
Leigh Alon
  Johns Hopkins University School of Medicine
Lillian Hsu
  Paul L. Foster School of Medicine, Texas Tech University
Louis Perkins
  Indiana University School of Medicine
LynnMarie Jarratt
  University of New Mexico School of Medicine
Manali Sapre
  Icahn School of Medicine, Mount Sinai
Manuel A. Fierro
  University of California, Davis School of Medicine
Margot Manning
  Harvard Medical School
Maria Fazal
  Johns Hopkins University School of Medicine
Mark Parry
  Paul L. Foster School of Medicine, Texas Tech University
Mary McGrath
  The Ohio State University College of Medicine
Matt Daly
  University of California, Los Angeles School of Medicine
Melissa Huddleston
  Paul L. Foster School of Medicine, Texas Tech University
Melody Fang
  Rosalind Franklin University of Medicine
Meriam Ben Hadj Tahar
  Stritch School of Medicine, Loyola University
Michael Angela Omongos
  City University of New York School of Medicine
Michaela O'Neill
  Stritch School of Medicine, Loyola University
Michelle Nosratian
  Albert Einstein College of Medicine
Mohammed Mustafa
  Albany Medical College
Molly Brady
  University of Arizona College of Medicine, Tucson

Monica Joglekar
   Geisinger Commonwealth School of Medicine
Naomi Cole
   Dartmouth Medical School
Natalie Neale
   Perelman School of Medicine, University of Pennsylvania
Nicola Feldman
   Icahn School of Medicine, Mount Sinai
Nicole Goldberg-Boltz
   University of Arizona College of Medicine, Tucson
Nikhil Bellamkonda
   University of California, Los Angeles School of Medicine
Peter Azzam
   Loma Linda University School of Medicine
Prasanti Ravipati
   Drexel University College of Medicine
Rachel Dokko
   Keck School of Medicine, University of Southern California
Rachel Truong
   University of Central Florida School of Medicine
Reagan McKendree
   University of Florida College of Medicine
Rissa Zudekoff
   University of Arizona College of Medicine, Tucson
Russyan Mark Mabeza
   University of California, Los Angeles School of Medicine
Samiksha Annira
   Carver College of Medicine, University of Iowa
Sara Khan
   Albany Medical College
Sarah Mukhtar
   Sidney Kimmel Medical College, Thomas Jefferson
   University
Shilpa Ghatnekar
   Tufts University School of Medicine
Shonit N. Sharma
   Carle Illinois College of Medicine, University of Illinois at
   Urbana-Champaign
Stephanie Tu
   Yale School of Medicine
Stephen Politano
   The Ohio State University College of Medicine
Teresa Veselack
   Stritch School of Medicine, Loyola University

Tiffany M. Nguyen
 University of Central Florida College of Medicine
Virali Shah
 Albany Medical College
Vivek Shah
 University of California, Los Angeles School of Medicine
Yuwen Cheng
 Renaissance School of Medicine, Stony Brook University
Zoe Brown
 Stritch School of Medicine, Loyola University

CPSIA information can be obtained
at www.ICGtesting.com
Printed in the USA
LVHW110525120522
718496LV00006B/245

"*Diary of a Med Student* helps us understand that we are not in this alone, and we are all more connected than we may think."
- SAUD SIDDIQUI, MD | Co-Founder of *SketchyMedical*

"An encouraging reminder that the honesty and transparency we hope for in our patients should be shared by us and each other. No one is alone in their journey!"
- DUSTYN WILLIAMS, MD | Founder of *Online Med Ed*

"A beautiful collection of stories about medicine. The heartfelt voices of these medical learners are touching and inspiring."
- JASON RYAN, MD | Founder of *Boards and Beyond*

• • • • • • • • • • • • • ● ● ● ● ● ● • • • • • • • • •

From the earliest stages of our medical training, we experience unforgettable moments with our patients - inspiring, traumatic, joyful, and sometimes even humorous events. Too often, as doctors-in-training we talk about the suffering or recovery of patients, ignoring our own emotions after these events, letting them passively shape us until we dig ourselves into an abyss of burn out and resentment.

This is a book created by medical students, for medical students, doctors, pre-med students, and their loved ones to look backward, forward, and laterally on the wonderful world of medical school. This book offers a space to reflect on our emotions, process their meaning, and share them as tales of sorrow, humor, joy, or inspiration, told from the perspective of medical students writing in a diary.

While the act of sharing emotion is itself therapeutic, reading these emotional challenges that we can all relate to is unifying and comforting, providing us with insight through the lessons conveyed in the light of a variety of feelings. Let this book spark a powerful domino effect of change in medical education: in the way we teach physicians to create a safe space for inner reflection and expression of emotion to ultimately enhance physician wellness.

• • • • • • • • • • • • • ● ● ● ● ● ● • • • • • • • • •

Daniel Azzam &
Ajay Nair Sharma
are MD/MBA Candidates at the UC Irvine School of Medicine. As Founders and Editors-in-Chief of *Diary of a Med Student,* they are humbled to share a collection of heartfelt stories from students across the nation.

ISBN 978-1-0879-0697-3
51299

9 781087 906973

www.diaryofamedstudent.com